Dipping in to the Duchy.

Wild Swimming in Cornwall plus many other areas of interest for your Kernow experience.

Chryseis

ISBN: 9781980289180

DEDICATION

We dedicate this to all those with the courage to try a Wild Swim and of course to all who helped with the making of this book most especially Katherine Moseley and Jenny Scott.

CONTENTS

Dipping in to the Duchy

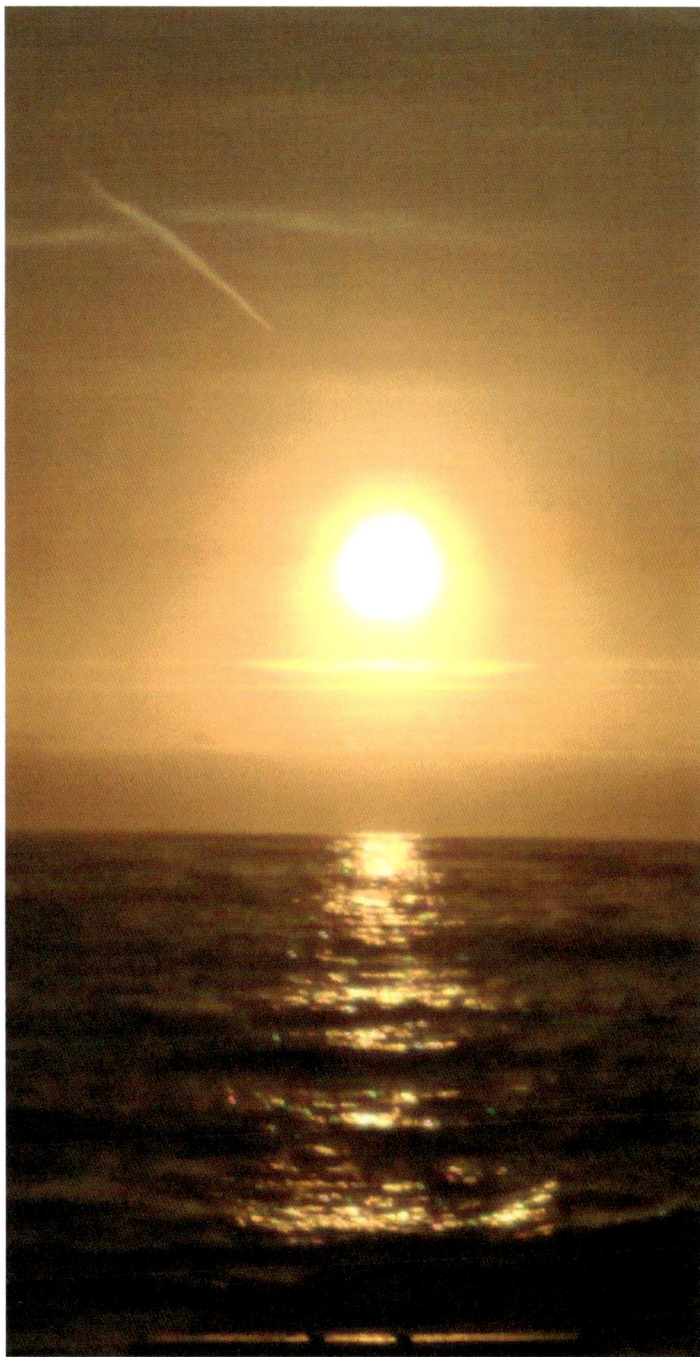

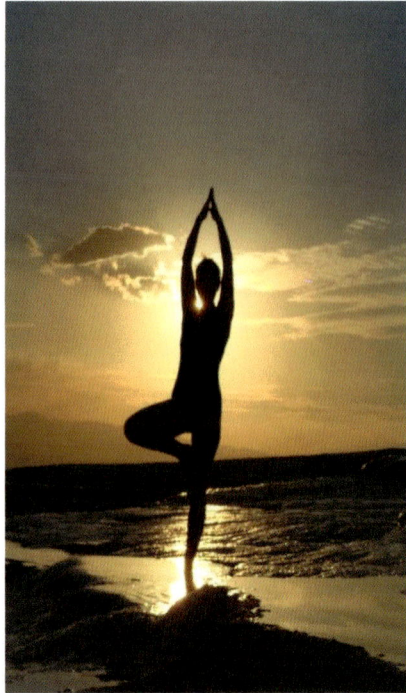

"Namaste or "Alright?"
"Yeah, you?"
"Yeah."

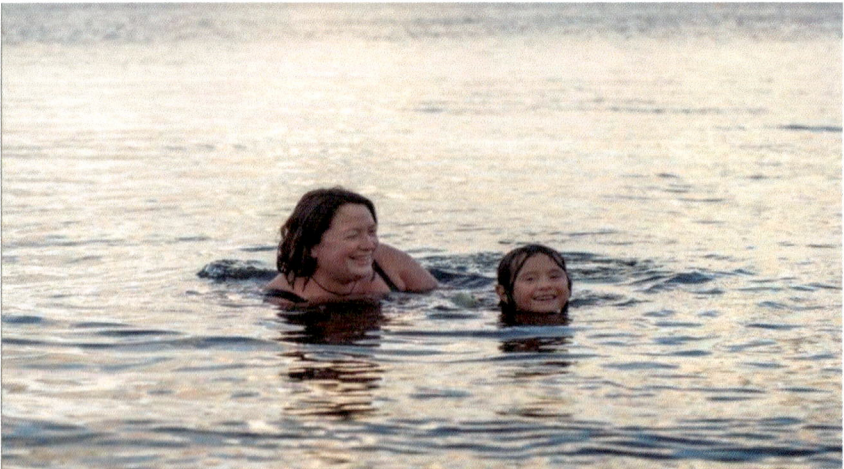

Picture courtesy of Sally Mitchel.

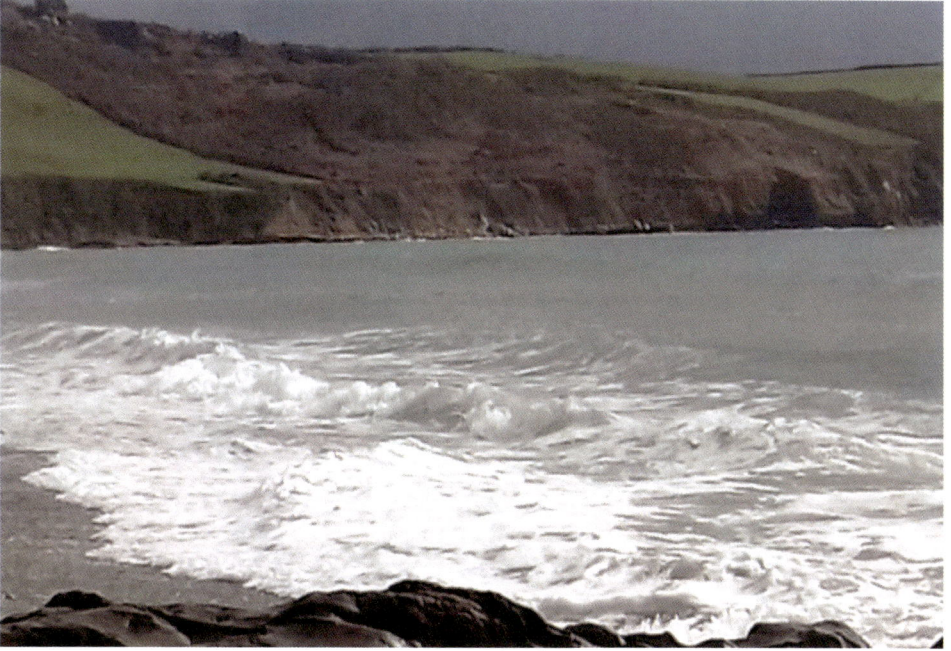

Mevagissey Bay looking east.

DEDICATIONS AND ACKNOWLEDGMENTS.

Here's a big shout out to all those who accused us of being mad and crazy, this further encouraged a joyous and life enhancing hobby.

Special thanks to Katherine, Morgan, Rowan, Megs and Tilly Moseley and Lily for coming out to play with us. To Jenny Scott for encouraging more Swims and helping edit the book, to Dale Buck for his patience taking over the homestead when Chrys dropped everything to go Swimming and for additional ideas. As well as Claire Tregunna for the finale proof read and D.Jenkins for IT support and encouragement.

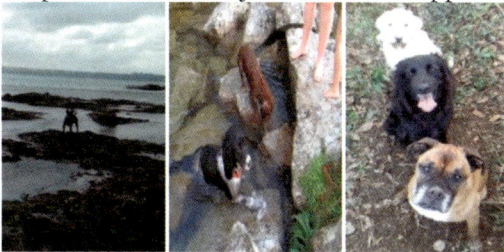

Cameo roles played by Scoobie, Sally and Harley.

1. Introduction: How we suggest using this book. The Who, the When, the Where, the How (The must read if Dipping) and the Why!?

Hello and welcome 'warmly', or possibly post a Swim, coldly but fully 'alively', to our first book in the series of places to Wild Water Swim in Cornwall. Here we have a selection and description of several of our favourite places, primarily in the South of Cornwall. We will use the Cornish name for Cornwall; Kernow, interchangeably to make you more familiar and comfortable with the Celtic name ☺

Each chapter does what it says 'on the tin' and includes the place name, a little geology, local information, and any additional instructions or material that we consider you may need or be interested in. Therefore, you can choose to follow a route incorporating all the included venues, perhaps more of your own along the route, or simply pick individual sites to try out and see just how much you love it ☺

We recommend this book as a guide and a source of local information when visiting these special named places and for extending your Kernow knowledge more generally☺

We have included an abundance of information about Cornwall for those who have interests in the fuller picture of this beautifully exquisite, 'characterful' county out on Britain's far west point☺

We think this may be good for conversation starters, teaching tools, pub quizzes, or simply for those who wish to know more. Perchance as a learning activity for the car, coach, train, tent, caravan, B&B or hotel when embedded in Cornwall, or to reflect upon a visit here when back up country ☺

There is space at the back for notes or sketches or maybe for lists of places to visit; we have abbreviated those recommended mid-text as ATL (Add To List)☺

We would like to suggest *that all taking part in Swimming or those accompanying Swimmers do please read most of chapter 2; especially the Health and Safety advice.* Although one may think they know it, in our minds; it's always useful to be reminded of safety measures☺

Feel free to skip and ignore the sections you (may) see as irrelevant, or in a polar opposite way (yeah, it can feel that cold) feel free to engage, underline and turn page corners for future information remembering and sharing☺

We could of course have expanded on; the history; the flora and fauna, and so many other equally fascinating areas. We have chosen to limit the book's scope otherwise the additional encyclopedic knowledge would not make your book easy to carry in already stuffed backpacks☺

We've added a collection of pictures of a variety of fauna pictures taken in Kernow for interestingness as well as a metaphor to suggest that we, as Wild Swimmers, are as different from each other as these creatures. Being passionate lovers of wildlife we have chosen to donate 25% of the books profits to the Cornwall Wildlife's Trust Marine Strandings Network. We apologize in advance to those who already clean beaches and tidy their own and others' messes for the frequent reminders to pick up any litter found whilst Dipping in to the Duchy☺

Have fun, enjoy, be safe and dive both metaphorically into the book and literally if you find it clear and have tested for water depth! ☺

THE WHO: US.

It didn't take long after Katherine and Chrys met for them to take a plunge. The sea and all its 422 miles of coastline are always close when on this Cornish promontory. One is never over 20 miles from the sea and mostly far closer. Both of us are women of a 'certain age', Chrys being decidedly more certain than Katherine! With this certainty there often comes a renewed joie de vivre, alternatively known as a second childhood; no shame or embarrassment to be felt, alongside a confidence and revived enthusiasm for adventure and play.

Katherine had holidayed at the exquisite little beach of Portmellon as a child. She now lives there with her husband, their two girls; Morgan and Rowan, and their two dogs; Megan and Tilly.

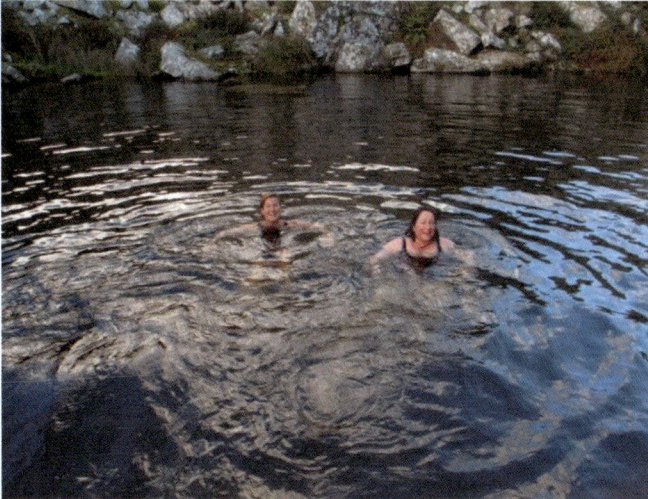

Chrys moved down from the somewhat oppressive London to the delightful, airy freedom of Pentewan with her ol' dog Lily, and the self proclaimed 'hardy women' met at a social event. Chrys's original intention, rather pretentiously was to write; 'pretentiously' as it seems that so many people come to Cornwall to be an 'artiste' of some persuasion and varying calibres. Chrys was also doing extreme fostering at the time, and even her young fostered London Town guest loved the regression and the healthy recreation they partook in during Wild Swimming sessions. This included a New Year's Day Wild Swim in the sea at Portmellon; yes, the airwaves were ripe with voluminous expletives and this was the women!

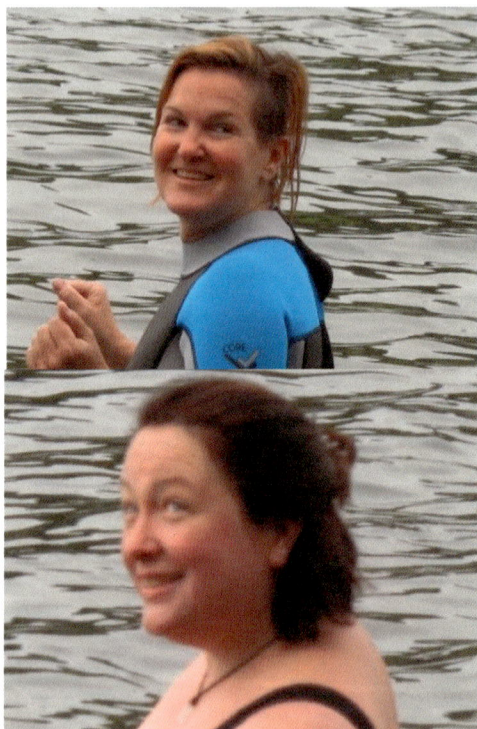

Neither of us are currently overt sports persons or competitive thus the adventures were for fun, health, exhilaration and thrills. We did not do miles and miles of water strokes. On occasion Chrys did her scream, yell and swear (profusely), dunk, several fast strokes and run back to dry land to wrap up warm and find a soothing hot drink! It must be noted; the more one swims in cold water, the easier it gets and the length of time immersed increases. Conversely the amount and volume of the expletive verbalizations reduces!
Both of us, some people may wish to note, follow a Vegan diet. We have interests in many other areas, for example Katherine rescues stranded seals

seasonally, and Chrys has a homestead that includes rescued battery hens. We are overt environmentalists, and we need to say this strongly and really accentuate the following: wherever you go, PLEASE take your own waste and belongings home, but also any other rubbish you find along the way. Yeah, we know the word 'hippies' is going through your mind!

If you take your canine companions with you, obviously take your biodegradable 'poo' bags, and check the time of year: many, especially south coast beaches, do not allow dogs from Easter until October. North Coast beaches seem far more accepting of our canine companions all year round. Cornwall has 53 beaches that permit dogs all year, 81 restricted and 7 full bans!

THE WHO: YOU.

We believe you can be of any age and of any physical; mental; emotional and psychological ability. The proviso being that those of extreme ages, at either end of the spectrum, cannot so readily control their own body temperature. therefore they are of special concern with the cold or hot!. For these sections of society, we recommend the warmer season, enjoying shorter dips and/or using really good protective covering! Accessible Countryside for Everyone (ACE) has a list of Cornish beaches accessible to the physically disabled. Not all beaches they reference have a ramp that reaches the sea at all tides, so it would be best to check first.

Thus if you can Swim, float, be held, or simply safely dunk under to get the 'cold water effect', we highly recommend you give it a try. We believe you're gonna love it☺

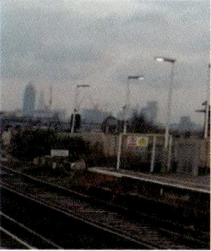

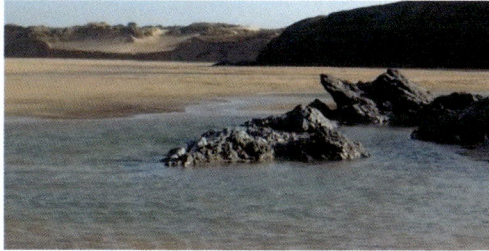

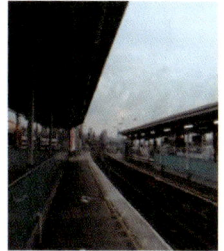

We know where we'd rather be☺

Thus far, the only genuine reason we have found for not participating in a Swim is fear. Obviously, fear is a perfectly acceptable emotion in relation to this challenge. To quote the title of a rather famous book, we still suggest that you; 'Feel the Fear and Do It Anyway' (S. Jeffers). Conquering fear is extremely life affirming, and when you get to the WHY section below, you'll see SO many other reasons, whoever you are, why we think you should at very least TRY IT!

See if you can name which species travelled here by their own accord and are thus Kernow maids and boys; which were bred here, and which imported? You and/or children may wish to write the genre and species in the spaces thus really owning your book. Perhaps list any fauna you find not pictured here or, extend this into a project that gathers the names and pics of flora too?

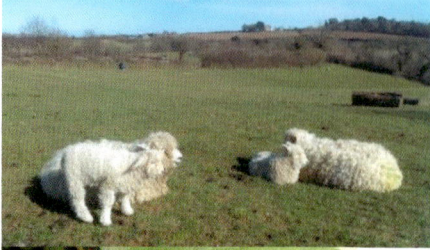

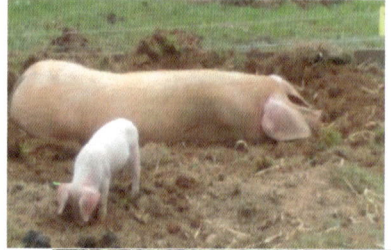

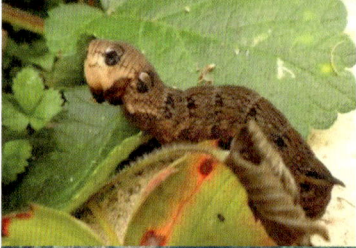

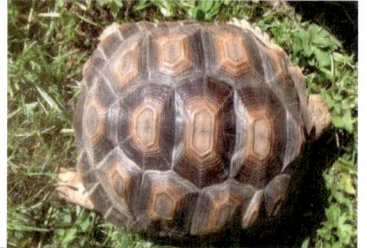

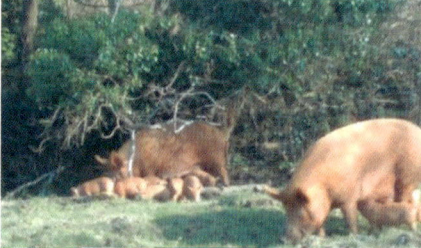

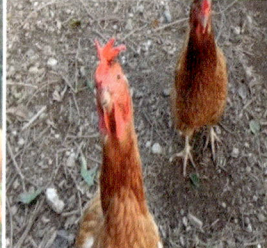

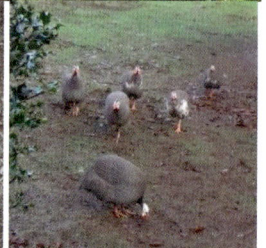

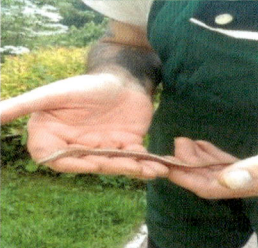

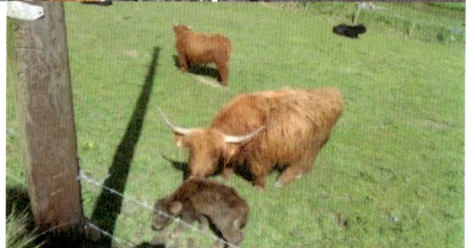

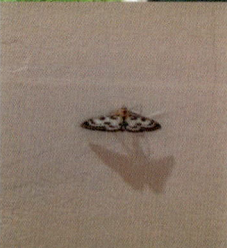

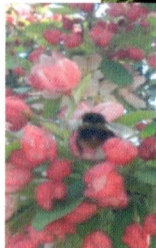

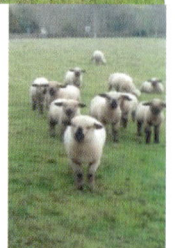

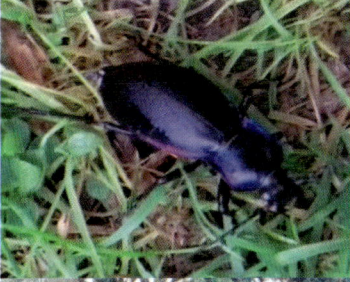

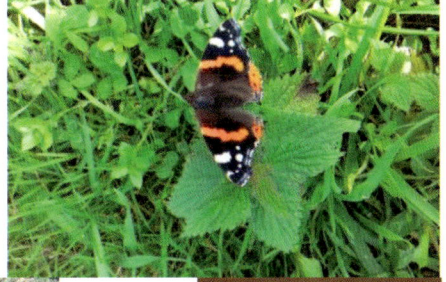

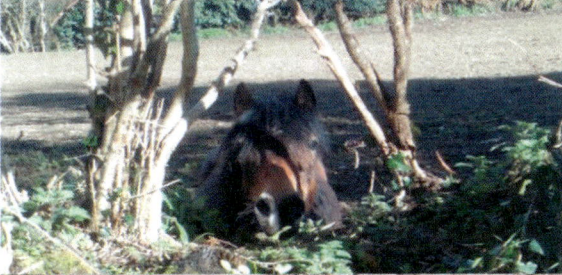

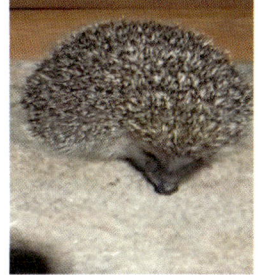

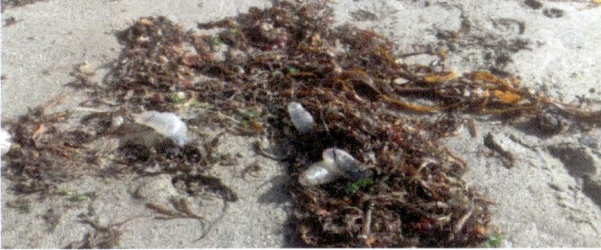

An extreme weather event bought what appeared to be colourful blown up prophylactics (if you don't understand this word then we'll say, for the younger reader: 'balloons'!) Extremely unusually they appeared in huge abundance in September 2017. This unceremonious stranding was of Portuguese Men of War (Physalia physalis). Even dead and plastic looking (and that's offensive enough) they can give a damn good sting! We never-the-less saw courageous surfers taking advantage of the unusually good south coast waves seemingly fearlessly whilst under threat of pain! The media news reports, and the Kernow grapevine, of this particularly noteworthy event had spread as a web. Like the strandings, the news had followed the most common sea currents; from the north around Land's End and up along the south coast. This pattern is repeated with the seal birthing too-Gweek Seal Sanctuary on the Helford River is worth a visit. (ATL).

It takes all sorts of flora and fauna to create a healthy eco-system and now it's time for us homo sapiens to help protect the ones we've started to destroy, and preserve those yet untouched☺ The Latin translates in to 'wise man'-may we suggest as a species we need to treat our natural environment rather more wisely adding in the life enhancing activity of Wild Swimming and we suggest you; Be More Seal!

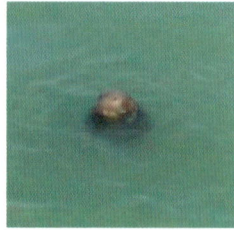

THE WHEN.

Katherine's children being home schooled, meant we took our adventures when we could; as often as we could; when the motivation and inspiration hit or when the sheer need to feel fully alive overtook us. We certainly only partook in daylight Swimming; while night time is of course a viable option, it comes with increased protective security advice.

The tides must first and fore mostly be considered. When the tide is out, the distances are further to walk, especially if the beach's angle is shallow extending the meterage to traverse. This is most important when returning from a Swim, as the coldness can feel rather harsh over a distance especially if ones' towels and snuggly coverings are far away. The often strong pull of the water can be an issue when the sea is retreating in other words; there's a heightened risk of being pulled out to sea as it goes out. Consequently we consider it safer to Swim as the tide is returning.

Tides times vary irregularly, and forward by between roughly half an hour to an hour per day in Cornwall. This is not the same everywhere; the changes are influenced by numerous convoluted and complicated factors to create different tide heights and thus distances to travel. The largest tide height variation was 6.31m and the lowest 0.9m.

One would need at least 'A' levels in Maths and Physics to calculate them. Let's simply say the main factors are astronomical and that one should always check: Websites, the little book with tide times sold at many retail outlets (see Pic), the local radio and TV stations. As well as the above sources, during the high season, most popular beaches and resorts display tide times along with wind strength, wave height, roughness, and even choppiness.

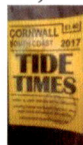

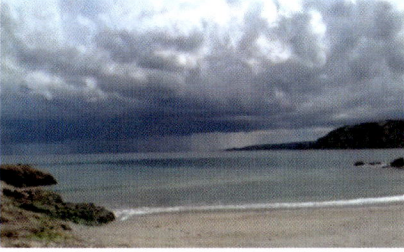
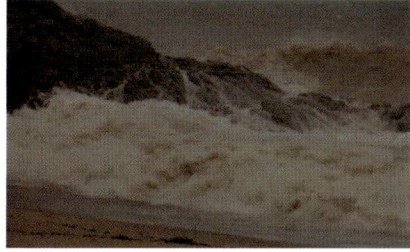

Pentewan on a bit of a rough and ready day-we can all relate and Pentewan trying to decide what mood it's going to be in☺

We would never suggest Swimming in the sea when it's raging with high waves, or even (unless properly equipped) lake or quarry Swimming when the temperatures can create serious health hazards such as freezing eyes! Our editor does Wild Swimming in lakes 'up country' and has to wear protective eye covering goggles for this very reason! Of course, a fabulous reason for goggles is also to be able to see and explore beneath the watery surface.

Please be aware that the weather changes rapidly in Cornwall: being a promontory into the sea, we receive the prevailing westerly winds. This means we most commonly get our weather from the Atlantic before the rest of the mainland does. We personally suggest; watching the skies, the animals and other homo sapiens in the area as additional guides to what information the TV, Radio and search engines may provide. Cornwall with its extreme landscapes has numerous micro-climates; if one is inland on a south facing slope, it can feel really hot and look calm but on arriving at the beach destination, with the hoped for smooth sea, things may not be as you had hoped to find.

THE WHERE.

The sea Swims in this 'first in the series' book are in our local St Austell and Mevagissey Bays, many other bays are of course available. It is a stunningly beautiful, generally, south facing coastline. Cornwall has nearly 220 beaches in total to choose from and almost one third of Cornwall is a designated 'Area of Outstanding Natural Beauty' this means, thank goodness, that it has the same protection as a National Park!

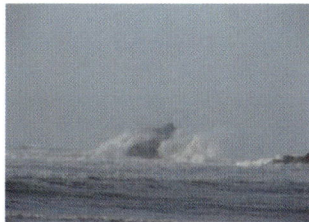

Crantock Bay-near Newquay- looking at the Celtic Sea in a real fury

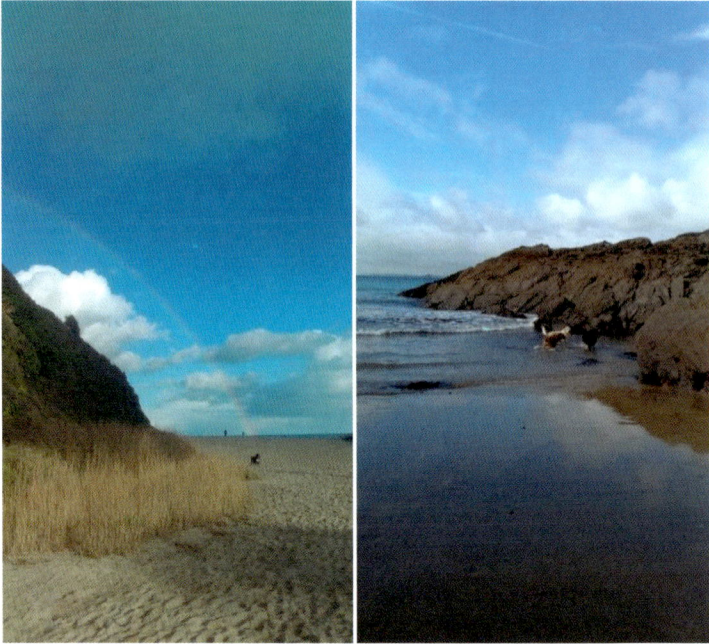

One does so hope for the rainbow and then the calm ☺

The North Coast of Cornwall has a tendency to be wilder, windier and therefore often much wavier. The North Coast is familiar for its famously reknowned beaches including; St Ives, Perrenporth and Newquay which make for wonderful Swims and may be included in later books! It must be noted that these areas, of course are most known for surfing due to the Atlantic waves. During the summer high season, a lot of beaches are divided between activities, but not out of season. This must be taken into consideration. Chrys's biggest fear, when she incompetently and inelegantly tries to surf, is that she may decapitate a swimmer as she hurtles speedily towards them unable to steer!

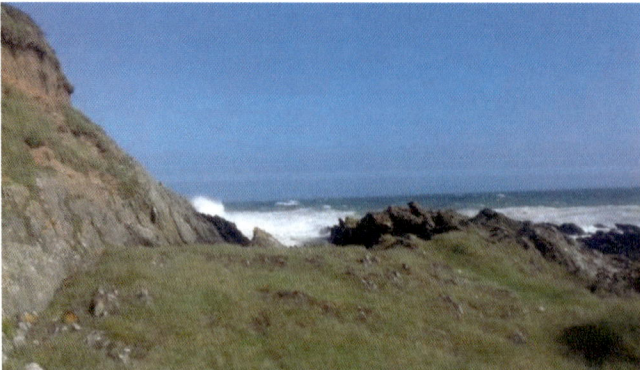

The South Coast interestingly has the better train connections as well as two of the most familiar names in tourist spots: The world-renowned Eden Project and The Lost Gardens of Heligan.

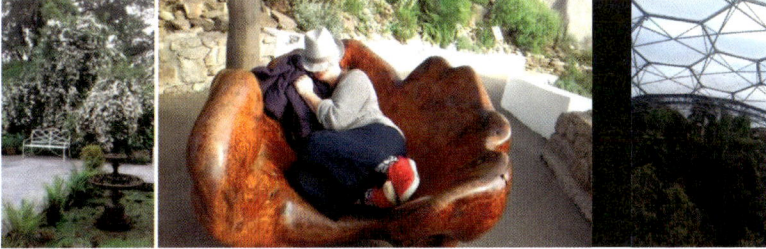

Places perchance for quiet contemplation within the Lost Gardens of Heligan or to sleep at The Eden Project after a swim☺

THE HOW; Including Safety Suggestions.

Katherine's 'how' is rather faster than Chrys's 'how'. Chrys has formulated a theory that; slow and steady immersion helps cool the blood as it pumps its way around the body, thus the top half the body (mind and soul) is not so shocked in comparison with the bottom half of the body (mind and soul). Thus it's not as harsh as it may have been getting one's shoulders under. This method also helps avoid the Cold Water Shock Effect that includes sharp intakes of rapid breathing, the heart working harder as blood vessels constrict and a gasp that could result in swallowing water if below the surface. This physical and involuntary response is short lived but can be dangerous for those with heart conditions. The slow styley can also give comfort when other people appear so much braver than one self. This immersion is additionally advised for the howlers; squealers; clenchers; screamers and swearers, as it gives more opportunity for these alternative spectacularly healthy and life enhancing self expressionistic behaviours! Those close by however may not feel so 'life affirmed', and they may even start quoting Satre's: "Hell is other people" as the cold water hits parts these temperatures rarely reach. The vocalisations tend to be exclamations that can become effusive and undoubtedly voluminous. We do so delight in philosophy and since we do have free reign to write anything we want in our own and now your book, here we go again with the 'maybe not at all relevant information'……………………………………………………………………..

"Hell is other people" is a quote from Sartre's play entitled; *No Exit*. Satre was a French existential philosopher-nought much more existential, and a reminder of being fully alive and therefore fully existing than Wild Swimming! *No Exit* is a play that illustrates the difficult coexistence of people: the play delineates the fact that others and their gaze is what alienates, and locks one in a particular kind of being and in turn deprives one of freedom. We don't want anyone deprived of anything, therefore we add to the Health and Safety section here: to always make sure you have *an exit* before entering any body of water. Chrys translates; "Hell is other people", perhaps more simply as freewill being taken away by 'other things' such as societies, cultures and civilization's norms and expectations having dominance over our own choices. As Chrys is a therapist hoping to support people's journey out of existential despair; she therefore likes to balance this "Hell is other people" with "Heaven is other people". Freewill, she suggests would undoubtedly be rather a bore, a little sultry and certainly unentertaining without other people or beings; 'Nuff said.

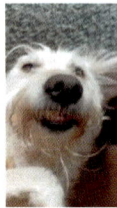

A smile would not be so satisfying without us to see and appreciate. We mostly walked barefooted to the closest Swim sites thus demonstrating a rather inelegant toe placing ballet move. Our gait was transformed from the obviously usual elegance, to this highly entertaining mode due to the surfaces being uneven; rocky; stony; pebbly and/or cold and sandy. The other sites, we drove as close to as possible and sometimes we remembered our sea shoes! Most Swims except for Bodmin and Trelissick, recommended here, have close-by parking spaces though very often limited, especially in the tourist season. This is primarily the 6 week school holiday time but also the period from the Easter season with a lot of Germans, and the 'tea and pee' brigade to mid Autumn. 'Tea and pee' is a saying referring to the coaches of mostly elderly folk who arrive, relieve themselves, refill with part of the daily tea quota, and then re-climb aboard their trusty coaches rarely to be seen again.
We wear our Swimming costumes in the warmer seasons, and maybe add long sleeved t-shirts and leggings when it's a bit cooler and then Chrys, in her less hardy and more wimpish way, dons a half wet suit for the extra chilly Swims. She also now wears highly recommended beach shoes because of having been stung once by a Weever fish; Echiichthys vipera.

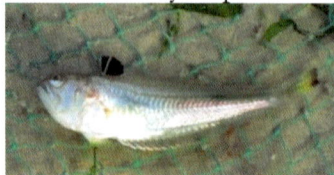

So! Beware of a small (10cm or so in legnth) sand coloured fish that spends most of its time buried under the sea bed with just a horribly venomous dorsal fin, awaiting the unaware bare footed human sand walkers. Woe betide a bather who steps upon a buried fish! The pain is excruciating as the spines embed into the human's flesh where the fish inserts its venom. Chrys forgot her sea shoes at Porthpean late 2018 and experienced it-it felt like standing on glass but with no blood or sign of injury. Suffering, yelling and moaning are at their most intense for the first two hours when the foot goes red and swells up. It then feels numb until the following day with irritation and pain that may last for up to two weeks! If the spine breaks off into the foot, it will cause discomfort until it is removed!

The *good news* is that if one gets the injured area in to, as hot as possible, water very soon then the pain retreats quickly. The heat kills the poison. OUCH! Now on with some more warnings before you hear the delights; "The brighter the light the deeper the shadow" an' all that!

Safety and Health; Rules and Regs!

General Swim Advice.

It goes without saying that there is always a risk associated with Wild Swimming-the giveaway being the 'Wild' aspect in the name. One's competence at Swimming per se has to be taken into account especially at the more 'extreme' sites of adventure.

> ➢ Don't drink alcohol or misuse substances.
> ➢ Don't Swim alone.
> ➢ Keep an eye out on the weather so that you know both tide times and if heavy rainfall is due or has fallen recently.
> ➢ If you suffer from any medical conditions, think about some of the locations for example in a quarry, the water can be much colder than you'd expect.
> ➢ Those with heart difficulties may wish to consult their GP or medic before considering this as a pastime.
> ➢ Make sure you do your own continuous risk assessment each time you go to a site in case the landscape or environment has changed since the writing of this book.
> ➢ Consider what you wear-not all locations will be happy with 'au naturel,' and a costume will not protect against the colder temperatures; a half wetsuit will restrict movement but allow for a longer dunk. A full wetsuit or dry suit may not only restrict movement but also be a nuisance to put on and remove. A dry suit may also 'dull'

the excitement and the thrill of the adrenalin rush, the fight or flight primal reaction to being immersed. (A trick to taking a 'wetsuit' off more easily, if you have succumbed, is to do so in the water).

➤ Remember to keep cuts and wounds covered with waterproof plasters if you are concerned.

➤ Avoid contact with blue–green algae (cyanobacteria) which is renowned for harming dogs and many others species.

➤ Where there is a possibility of animal urine as a contaminant in the water, for instance near sewage outlets or certain water runoff areas, please be aware of Leptospirosis commonly known as Weil's Disease. Weil's is often associated with rats, but can also be transferred from other sources. Numerous people contract the illness and have only mild reactions to this bacterial infection. If you feel ill between 3 days and 3 weeks after a Wild Swim do consult a GP as it can be life threatening for some people.

➤ To repeat ourselves; please try never to Swim alone and do keep a constant watch on weak Swimmers especially as there is a tendency for this experience to become addictive.

➤ Never jump into water you have not thoroughly checked for depth and obstructions.

➤ Always make sure you know how you will get out before you get in. *No exit* must never be an option.

➤ Don't get too cold. We recommend a warm up with exercise and warm clothes both before and after a Swim. Some medics (and Chrys) suggest going in slowly to stop muscles spasming especially on hotter days as the shock comes from the temperature variations between air/skin and water.

➤ Cold Water Shock is a natural body response and completely out of your conscious control. The body makes you gasp an in-breath and one's heart rate increases rapidly; so never put your mouth under water straight away. Breathe steadily and allow the Swimming to warm you up. Acclimatisation is highly recommended to avoid this; slow and steady repeated immersions, lengthening in time as one adapts.

➤ Wear footwear if you can especially if you are 'coasteering' as part of the fun.

➤ Never wave your arms in fun. Watchers need to know if there is a difficulty. Although it appears that one cannot usually demonstrate the usual signs of fear when close to drowning! Perhaps consider having an accessible whistle with you is also a good piece of kit.

➢ Hypothermia is an ever present fear with Cold Water Wild Swimming. If you shiver in the water GET OUT and warm up quickly. You can always try the finger touching test-each digit to the thumb, and if this is awkward or unattainable again GET OUT and warm up.

➢ On the above point Chrys has Reynaud's Syndrome (where the blood supply to extremities is affected by the cold) she therefore keeps hands and feet covered during the colder Swims. You may wish to follow this practice.

➢ If you get cramp then float on the water and shout for help. Be aware that cramping is a sign of hypothermia or tiredness and it is suggested that you get to dry land ASAP.

➢ Always stay hydrated as you would with any physical activity. If you get really good and confident at Swimming as an exercise that will deplete your reserves, and this may not be noticeable when in the water, and busy smiling, and having fun. (Saying that; an US Army research group that there is very little harm caused by dehydration in cold weather!)

Sea Swim Advice.

❖ Be aware that the variation in tide heights and, thus speed of the incoming and outgoing waters. The range from the 'astronomically-influenced' tide is from roughly 6 meters at the highest to at around 1 meter at the lowest. (These do not include variables such as tidal surges created by storms and run off post heavy rain). Interestingly the highest spring and neap tides (when the sun and moon are aligned in the sky versus being on opposing sides of the Earth) are slightly lower. Do ponder the difference of roughly 5 meters height of water and its resultant voluminous effect!

❖ A rip tide-or current- is most Swimmers' worst nightmare, as the undersea channel pulls the water and thus anything in it out to sea, usually pretty fast. The difficult, but necessary action is to Swim *across it*, not ever trying to go against it, as this WILL NOT work.

There are some clues to seeing if a rip tide is present on a beach.

1. A still section of water being noticeable in rougher waves.

2. Debris such as seaweed drifting out in a line and

3. Darker water where the stronger current may have stirred up more sand.

<u>Inland Swim Advice.</u>

o It is not considered wise to Swim in canals, locks or urban rivers. South West Water disallows Swimming in reservoirs

o There are numerous additional dangers if one considers Swimming in flood water so we categorically say; "Don't."

o Conversely be cautious of water quality during droughts.

<u>Specialist Equipment Ideas.</u>

✓ Watch out for boats on any navigable river and it is advisable to wear a coloured Swim hat so you can be seen.

✓ Another vital piece of recommended equipment is a colourful float. It won't keep you afloat but you will be more visible.

✓ A whistle may also be a good idea.

So hopefully we haven't put you off with the 'rules and regs', and hope we're not sounding like we are collaborating with the fear culture that we live in. The safety advice should be read and memorized or re-read prior to dunking. Then it's time to get on and enjoy life and have a Wild Swim. To boost your life experience choice as well as to re-confirm your decision to Wild Swim now we suggest reading the WHY; just below☺

THE WHY.

The above H&S was obviously extensive and thorough but, as we said, we may have added to the somewhat natural instinct and, the culturally promoted fear of adventure, so please read this section fully to regain the positivity...☺

We partake mainly because we love it, but there are also many beneficial health benefits to be gained from Wild Swimming. In particular, the cold water 'body shock' effect. This stimulates the flight and fight reaction of the Central Nervous System-thinking is turned off as energy is diverted away from non-essential processes including digestion. One's heart rate increases, blood pressure rises, blood is pushed to muscles (and elsewhere; see below)☺

Muscles are soothed of their aching by this form of invigoration; an internal massage! The full functioning of the blood working and flooding the body with adrenalin and cortisol a stress-reactive 'endo' (internal) hormone helps as an energetic stimuli. If one's bodily systems are slow or flat; a Cold Water Swim thoroughly helps lift mood and is medically recognised as being able to help relieve depression. The flight and fight reaction is healthy for short bursts but the Para-Sympathetic Nervous System should be allowed to kick in to; 'rest and digest' at the warming up stage of the Wild Swim☺

Nature and the Wild experience of nature and of being outdoors additionally and undoubtedly improve mental, social and emotional well being☺

A Cold Water Swim also boosts the immune system; white blood cell count is evidenced to increase significantly in studies☺

The water in Cornwall varies, during a normal year, between 7 and 15 degrees and only small pockets ever feel like 'a bath' as some commentators on the seas temperature have described the feel of the sea in warmer climes.☺

Anyone who has already tried Wild Swimming knows of that endorphin high that raises mood, can create elation, and of course excites and heightens the senses generally.('endo' meaning 'within' and the 'orphine' is a shortened 'morphine'). One can therefore understand why most people when they come out feel an almost addictive urge to dive back in, and how when one is immersed you often don't want to come out. It's easy to self deceive: for example Chrys had forgotten her gloves. She thus got out of the water this winter really quickly. She went on to convince herself that she was jealous of missing out on the waves-this had nothing to do with the real reasoning (OK, maybe a little to do with it) but what had actually happened was that her body had enjoyed the endorphin rush so much she immediately wanted more!☺

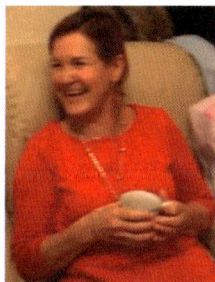

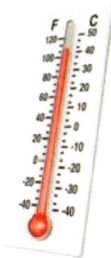

The afterglow with the warming drink.

The above are simply the immediate effects, below longer term benefits☺

The long-term impacts are well researched by NASA(National Aeronautics and Space Administration)demonstrating in research that over a 12-week period; repeated Coldwater Swimming leads to substantial bodily changes known as 'cold adaptation'. Blood pressure goes down and this in turn improves circulation☺

As the body heats up, one's blood is brought to the surface and the polar opposite happens when being cold: the blood gets sent to the organs. This increase in blood being pumped around your body helps flush your circulation, it will exfoliate your skin and flush impurities from it, thus helping your complexion and some say it will even reduce cellulite!☺

Another, we think, spectacular benefit is that one's cholesterol is lowered. This is because the lower temperature can burn twice as many calories as in warmer water. The body uses energy to keep warm thus reduces fat being deposited☺ Newborn humans and some adults have a brown fat whose primary function is that of thermoregulation. In fact it is 'heat generating' and is activated when exposed to cold. Bizarrely this fat can go on generating heat even after it's fed by sugars in the blood. (Whereas shivering stops after the blood sugar stores in the muscles are depleted). Not all of us have evolved to have this fat and it does take prolonged cold to stimulate it but, we hope we have, as it helps with the so often craved; weight loss☺

One needs to pee more when cold (cold dieresis). Therefore, if one is prone to water retention then a Cold Swim can stimulate your 'release', literally and metaphorically. So to pee or not to pee; that's our current question☺

Can you believe that there are even more physical health benefits to Cold Water Swimming? It inhibits blood clotting too which is another aspect of improved circulation. When one adds that; another physical manifestation of, Cold Water Swim, includes increasing fertility and libido (by increasing the production of testosterone and oestrogen in men and women, respectively), one wonders why we don't have government campaigns promoting it!☺

On a personal experiential level rather than actual research; Chrys has been experiencing hip pain and this recedes to nearly nothing after a Swim. The cortisol spike in the bodies flight and fight reaction helping, again, reducing pain reception. Again, this may vary from person to person, taste to taste, and mood to mood. Chrys has, post breast cancer treatment, had dry skin from the anti-oestrogen chemicals and now off it-even though as said; of a certain age; has greasier skin and hair again. Neither dry or greasy skins were affected by the sea water so the expectation of the sea drying skin seems to be a fallacy-it does though dry hair!☺

Salt consumption has had a bad name recently via the medical institutions and we live in a cultural climate that is critical of it; but it's minerals we definitely need. It's interesting to watch the revival of sales for 'healthier' salts such as Himalayan Rock Salt and the wonderful orange lights many of us more hippy types like to burn in the small hours☺

We know salt water is healing; as the compound sodium chloride is both a cleanser and an anti-inflammatory-this last factor being accentuated when combined with the water temperatures☺

We will add some facts again for those that may wish to indulge in some information-porn. In the open ocean salt is averagely 35 grams per litre which is roughly 3.5% of the waters entirety. Salt preserves food and we have taste buds especially to notice it so it may, in an homeopathic way, preserve us too! The skin is a carrier not a barrier so we will absorb salt. Katherine reminds

Chrys when Chrys is squealing at not greatly enjoying the feel of squishy and sometimes smelly seaweed, that we are also commonly absorbing additional nutrients during a Wild swim; such as magnesium (that is deemed great to help sleep). These components are free and available for our benefit in the water ready for our nourishment during a Sea Swim☺

Dissolved components in seawater

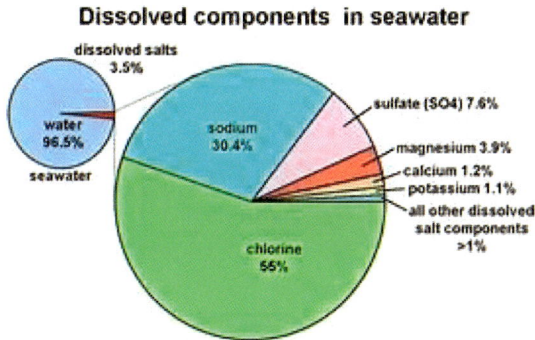

Sodium is an essential nutrient as it acts an electrolyte; which is what your body's cells use to maintain voltages across their cell membranes. As well as to carry electrical impulses; muscle contractions which one may certainly stimulate by entering for a Cold Wild Swim!

Salt has numerous other health benefits which we will simply list. To sprinkle or not to sprinkle, to dive in or not to dive in; that's your next question for today, but here's the encouraging list for this marvelous aspect of our world and our interaction with it…………………………………....☺

- Firstly and most basically it makes food TASTE better.
- It helps balance hormones.
- Salt combats cortisol-one of our stress hormones and can also help with thyroid issues.
- It also calms adrenaline this would strongly suggest that relaxation and sleep are therefore improved!
- Salt can speed up your metabolism.
- It can help heat production in the body-although we don't think you'll notice this benefit when Wild Water Swimming.
- Salt is an antihistamine
- It helps maintain stomach PH levels.
- Promotes blood sugar levels and some declare reduces the signs of aging-rejuvenation appears to be a real consequence of Wild Swimming per se!!

- Prevents muscle cramps-always good when going in to Cold Water as this may be a consequence of the indulgence!
- Promote vascular health as an addition to the already mentioned benefits of blood circulation with the temperature variation experienced with the swim!
- If added to potassium and water then it helps with blood pressure as well as the swim-where will we stop?
- Ok we'll stop here; a healthy percentage of salt intake actually increases physical energy.

Salts' mining has been carried out by us Homo sapiens since 5400BC where the first known European town was formed in current Bulgaria; named Solnitsata meaning salt works. Salt mining continues to this day primarily by the desalination of sea water. Salt was an early gold and used as a method of buying and selling. Its' value as a preservative helped us to keep food whilst travelling, therefore encouraging and promoting trade of other goods and ideas.

Salt has had powerful meaning for humans in religion, economy and culture since time immemorial.

Maybe it goes without saying that there is more salt in animal tissues, such as meat, blood, and milk, than in plant tissues. Nomads who subsist on their flocks and herds don't eat salt sprinkled as we may, those with a cereal and vegetable diet seem to need to sprinkle

As mentioned above; with the spread of settled and trading civilization, salt became one of the world's main commodities. Salt has been of extremely high value to many cultures including; ancient Hebrews, Greeks, Romans, Byzantines and Hittites. In the Middle East, salt was used to ceremonially seal an agreement, and the ancient Hebrews made a "covenant of salt" with God and sprinkled salt on their offerings to show their trust in him.

Conversely an ancient war practice was salting the earth: preventing plant growth until it. For instance; the Roman general Scipio Aemilianus Africanus was said to have ploughed over the city of Carthage with salt after it was defeated in the Third Punic War (146 BC). So the brighter the light the deeper the shadow encore! And there's us casually sprinkling it on our chips after a plunge in the sea without a second thought! FYI neither of us are on commission from the salt companies

Dipping in to the Duchy

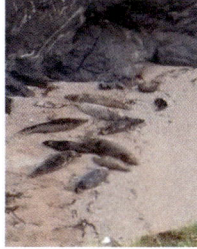

To summarize: Wild Water Swimming feels amazing and fabulous and tends to be free, and also does you enormous amounts of good. Not many other feel good experiences can make the same claim, and then after one is addicted it feels like something many of us 'have to do' not even 'choose to do'!

As a final point about mood enhancement and Wild Swimming; one necessarily has to be 'present' and 'in the moment' and fully aware in a mindful, or Buddhist practice sense of being. The sensations and the need to be fully focused take one away from other aspects of life, allowing the unconcious to get on and sort things out, whilst one conciously and literally have to 'let it go' so that you can get on with the Wild Swim in what are judged to be the UKs, and developed Europes best quality bathing waters:the Kernow seas.

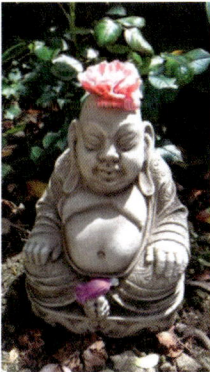

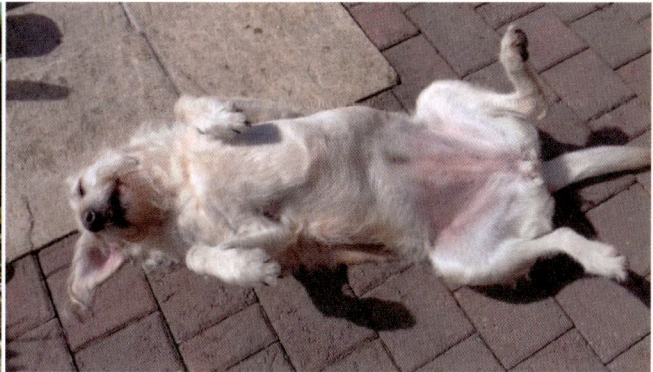

Guessing this guy is serene but not an experienced and practising Cold Water Swimmer! Sally demonstrating how we look and feel after excessive exertions in the Kernow waters ☺

Common words to describe the feeling after a Wild Cold Water Swim: refreshed, refuelled, revitalized, reinvigorated, released: all the 're' words. The implication being that; the 'performance of the new action brings back an earlier state of affairs' and therefore may we add rejuvenated. So leap in, and feel mentally, emotionally and physically younger!

Go ahead and jump or dive or slowly lower yourself in and feel your 're's'. RELEASE the pressure, breathe deeply in and then RELAX.

2. A Duchy Download; A bit of Geology; the Weather, including temperature variations of air and water; the demographics; the Economy; the Arts and Parking.

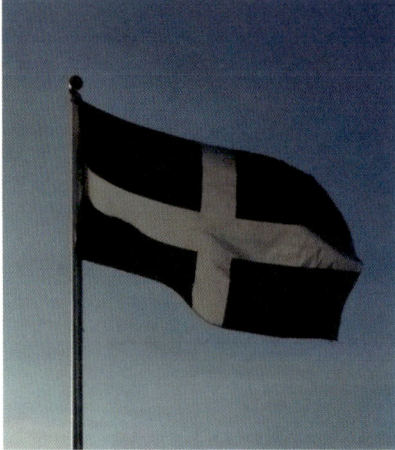

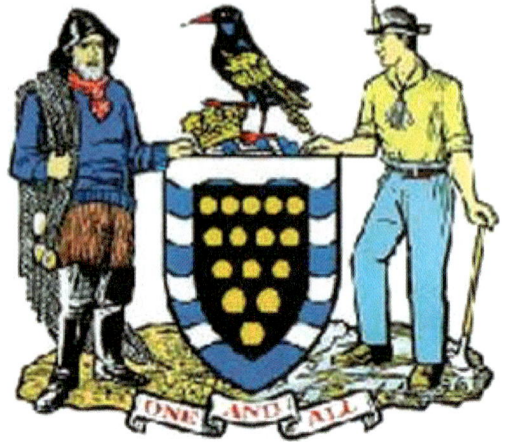

Cornwall or Kernow regularly flies the black flag with the white cross. This is humorously and commonly believed to be a pirate flag. Kernow is undoubtedly renowned for its historical pirate behaviours, including the hiding of bounty in its very available coves and caves, avoiding the guarded ports. An action that demonstrated Kernow's historical wish to avoid the control and taxation of Westminster still currently felt! (see Politics section; this Chapter). The Cornish are frequently characterized as non-conventional and their previous piratical import system reflects this fact! Chrys loves calling this outpost 'The Wild West' and not just for the available sites for Wild Swimming.

The Cornish Coat of Arms shows the 15 golden bezants (coins) apparently paid to the Saracens for the release of the kidnapped Duke of Cornwall- although this is not necessarily historically provable!

This chapter and the book title include the word 'Duchy' because Cornwall is not only Celtically named; Kernow but 'royally' named; the 'Duchy'; this jutting west-land being land 'owned' by the Prince of Wales. (He is also entitled the Duke of Lancaster; therefore there is a Duchy of Lancaster.)

Some more Kernow information porn:

In total Cornwall's land area is 135,000 acres; 3,563 km^2 or 1375.682miles^2 hemmed in by its 422 miles of coastline of which 158 achieve designated Heritage Status. Although, one tends to consider the North Coast as the Atlantic Ocean (and when considering a wider scale this can be seen as such).

Closer to land the body of water is called the Celtic Sea. The sea off the South Coast is, maybe more obviously, the English Channel.

Sea level is the lowest point (stating the bleeding obvious perhaps) and Brown Willy (giggles aside) is the highest point; a granite outcrop on Bodmin Moor. ATL and try to visit on non-mizzley days, it gets very boggy and we suggest keeping dogs on the lead as other animals roam free near here.

The largest lake is in far west in Cornwall, near Port Leven; named Lake Loe-more giggles emanating, wethinks. The longest flowing water is the Tamar River that borders Devon. It is 94 kilometres/58.4miles in length. The next longest is the Camel River at 50 kilometers/31.1 miles-both river basins and surrounding countryside offer enticingly delightful beauty, flora, fauna, walks and cycle paths. ATL

The seas are perhaps obviously a favourite attraction to both locals and emmets. (see Chapter 7). The waters are, generally fabulously clean and there are 6 Marine Conservation Areas namely; Polzeath, St Agnes, the Isles of Scilly, Fowey and Looe.

To repeat, and we feel this 'nag' does sadly needs much repetition: the problem is the beach litter, and washed up sea waste. The volume increases exponentially after storm surges, washing up shockingly large amounts of a variety of debris. Us 'gatherers' can fill up to 10 (biodegradable) dustbin liners in a few steps Our current geological era has sadly been referred to as 'the Plastic Age'. We strongly feel that we should try to keep that appellation for the landfill areas, and not the sea and ocean floors. So again, we repeat; please pick up rubbish after your selves and that of other less considerate and knowing persons! Thanks in advance ☺

Geology

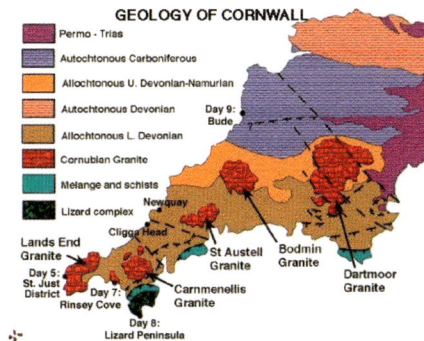

The above map is full of specialist and complex names; it does though give a good colourful image of the variation and divisions to be noted

A surprising factor in relation to the geology is that Cornwall has been known to experience intraplate tremors; earthquakes. Aargh! In 1814 there was a Cornish earthquake measuring 4.4 on the Richter scale, the epicenter being near Penzance. The rumbles increase in frequency the further West one goes in Kernow.

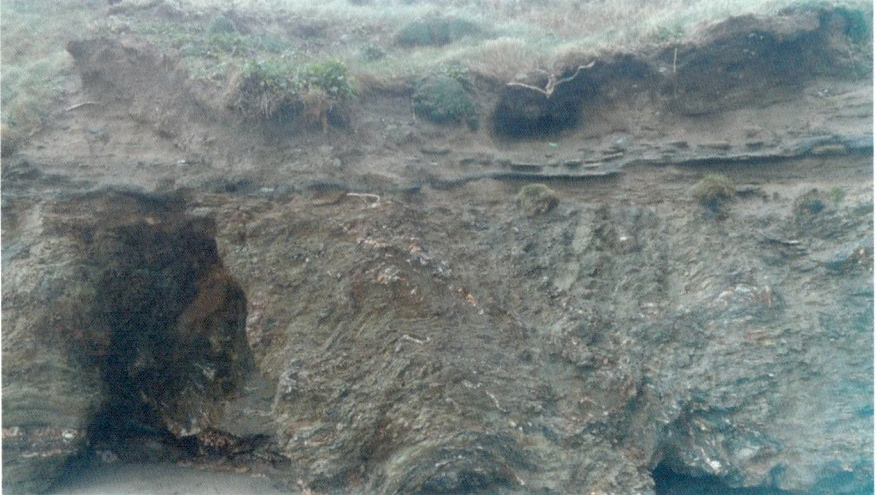

Curvature and clear stratification of the rocks to be seen at Pendower Beach on the Roseland Peninsula.

During the geological era namely the Paleozoic period, the world had two massive landmasses, named Laurasia and Gondwana. The tectonic 'plates' are constantly moving and adjusting as the surface landmasses shift on the melted molten magma below. Plate tectonics (Latin: pertaining to building) pushed the two together to make Pangea, when almost all the Earth's land surface joined as one. Pangea was surrounded by a global ocean called Panthalassa. This gigantic landmass was fully assembled by the Early Permian Epoch (some 299 million to 273 million years ago). The supercontinent began to break apart about 200 million years ago, during the Early Jurassic Epoch (201 million to 174 million years ago.) Very slowly over thousands of millennia, the plates formed the modern continents we now all recognize, know and love today. The reshaping of our world, of course created the Atlantic, Pacific and Indian Oceans as well as the smaller seas. This pre-verbal or written historical period would certainly have provided an extensive coastline, but there was very little evidence of fauna alive, or at least evolved enough to enjoy it; all was 'wild'; nothing tamed or civilized as yet.

Chrys did 'A' level Geography and, as is maybe already obvious, to this day a little obsessed with the subject. There are fabulous courses in Geology (and many more interesting subjects) available across Cornwall to expand the craving mind. For the here and now; the choice is yours to read or not to read, that is the current question!

OK here we go; the Paleozoic Geological Period lasted from 541 to 251.902 million years ago. It is subdivided into six shorter-term geologic periods (from oldest to youngest); the Cambrian, Ordovician, Silurian, Devonian, Carboniferous, and the Permian. The Paleozoic era was a time of dramatic geological, climatic, and evolutionary change.

The Cambrian Age witnessed the most rapid and widespread diversification of life in Earth's history; namely the Cambrian Explosion. During this huge timescale most modern classes of known species first appeared; fish, arthropods, amphibians and an abundance of primitive reptile subclasses. Also towards the end of the Paleozoic era, large and sophisticated vertebrates were dominant and the first modern tree appeared which was the conifer.

Life began in the ocean. Evolution and the search for more tempting resources eventually led exploration onto land. By the late Paleozoic, great forests of primitive plants covered the continents, many of which formed the coal beds of Europe and eastern North America. We have been fuelling ourselves with these furiously since the Industrial Revolution.

As we all know, we need to calm, in fact stop this consumption to waylay the already occurring climate changes on Earth. If there are any non-believers still about, we suggest recognising that; it's better to attempt to solve a problem and find out it's not real than it is to leave it and suffer the consequences with the discovery of its' reality; when changing behavior would be too late!

Now we have seen the bigger and much older picture, let us allow ourselves a little breather as we emerge to the here, if not quite fully in the now.

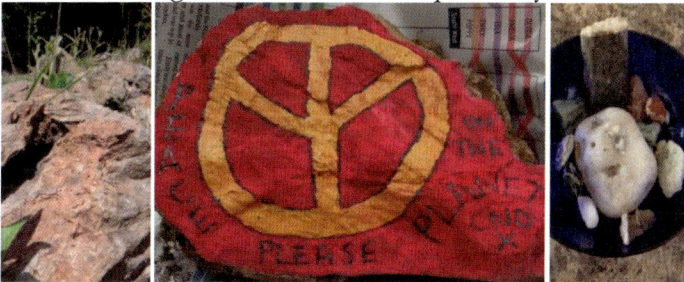

Some Kernow Rocks; one can certainly see the iron, feldspar, quartz and copper deposits. During 2018 a fad for painting rocks emerged; see Chrys' above. Give it a try (ATL)

Cornwall's igneous (volcanic) batholithic (literally meaning mass of granite rock), backbone of extrusive granite was created due to the mountain building era when the aforementioned massive landmasses (Laurasia and Gondwana) met and pushed against each other.

The granite was formed as the bubbling molten rock, called magma when below the surface and as lava once above. It forms deep within the mantle; which is beneath the continental and oceanic floors. The slow cooling, igneous rock is harder, and thus less easily 'weathered' than the surrounding 'killas'.

The bulk (literally) of Cornwall's geology is Devonian slate commonly called 'killas'; this is metamorphicised, sedimentary rock created when layer upon layer of deposited material changes its' composition due to heat and pressure. Killas is also from the original early land mass that the granite burst through or was uncovered due to weathering (see above). Killas actually underlies two thirds of Cornwall, as well as on and around Dartmoor in Devon. The land across the Tamar can be a little bit of a dirty word to some of the ol' Kernow Folk, the closest rival for resources always seems to create the in group/out group prejudices! ATL for discussion?

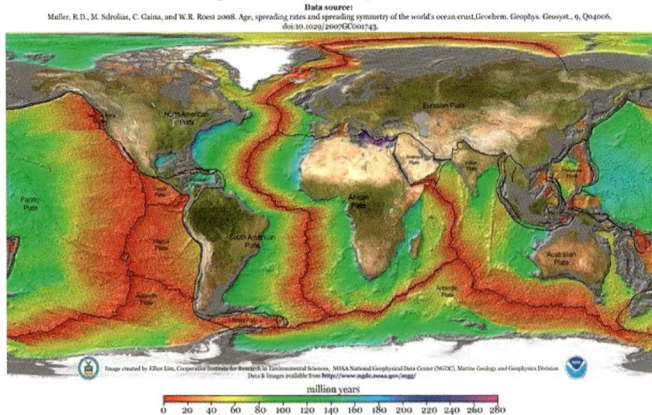

Age of Oceanic Lithosphere (m.y.)
Data source:
Müller, R.D., M. Sdrolias, C. Gaina, and W.R. Roest 2008. Age, spreading rates and spreading symmetry of the world's ocean crust,Geochem. Geophys. Geosyst., 9, Q04006.
doi:10.1029/2007GC001743.

Our planet with tectonic plates mapped; as we are, for now.

Granite remains our outstanding, sturdy Kernow backbone today. In a combination of science and poetry granite is known as the Rock of Ages; it can include all impurities, in more positive words; all elements, in larger and smaller quantities including Gold. Hydrothermal mineralization is heated water making changes; the polar opposite to the cooled water making changes to us as Wild Swimmers. This occurred within the granite creating the majority of Cornwall's mineral veins. These, at one time, provided up to half of the world's tin and copper, adding to the historical economic prosperity of Cornwall (and to a lesser extent Devon).

FYI One can visit a tin mine that sells Cornish Gold at Tolgus Mill near

Redruth.(ATL) not to be mistaken for the Cider or the Coffee named Cornish Gold.

Back to the general geology briefly, you may be pleased to hear; Pangea, as said, broke apart and travelled again around on the molten mantle. The plate's movement, splitting and travelling eventually bumped in to and placed Cornwall with the other British landmasses to create the familiar shape of our Isles.

As the covering softer materials were weathered away and removed by rivers, glaciers and wind over millions of years there was a consequential reduction in pressure and weight. Structural movement due to these changes created the folds, bends, fissures and cracks one can relish. Resulting in tors, valleys and all the delightful geology we are so privileged to see today.

Marsh and bogs form due to the impermeability of the granite (see Goldiggins Quarry Chapter 3.) in areas of heavy rainfall, consequential poorer soil. With the geologically late arrival of Homo sapiens', other species were tamed and fed on the natural flora instead of crop growing. Us vegans delight in seeing the beautiful mammals but are saddened by our 'use' of them; perhaps ATL to discuss!?

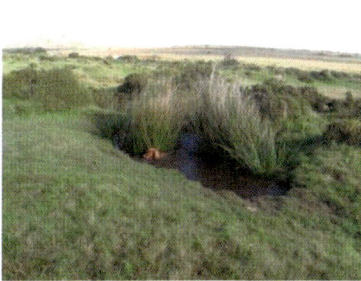

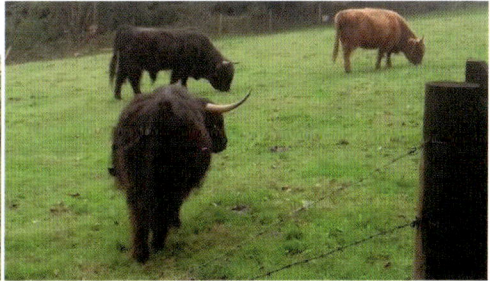

Boggy land mammals.

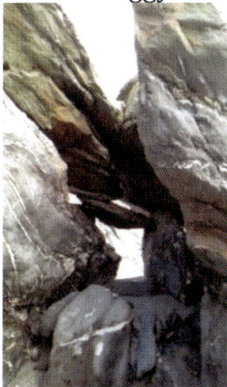

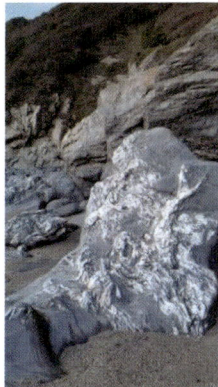

Vault Beach, over the headland from Gorran Haven.

Of lesser economic importance than the mineral impurities was, and is the stone itself; used for building and roofing. The largest single source in the county is the Delabole slate quarry. (One can do a tour here;ATL) It has provided high quality stone for at least six centuries.

Pentewan had its' own 'elvan' quarry produced a fine stone that could be easily carved; this was used in the construction of many of the Cornish Medieval churches. (See Chapter 5) Additionally, the Lizard peninsula gives rise to an unusual rock formed when the oceanic crust formed in the carboniferous age. Please see above colourful map.

We think you could perhaps research and explore, and try to find the variances in rocks whilst on your Cornish adventures- before, during or after braving your swims. Happy collecting and questioning which is which?

Weather.

We believe most of us fantasize that Cornwall's summers are complete with long, hot, hazy dreamy days, especially when one sees the more temperate plants that can grow here.

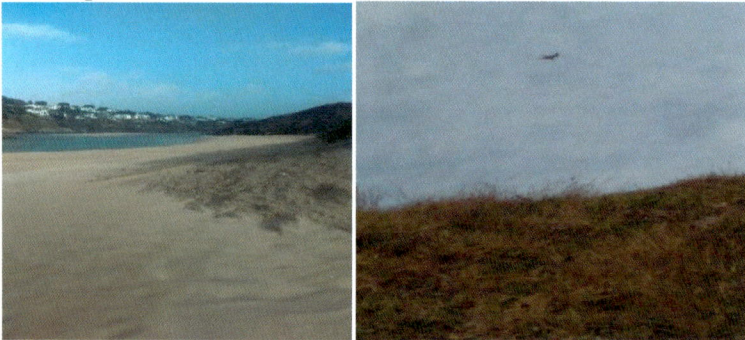

The Gannell near Newquay, and a buzzard above the cliffs at Mevaggissey.

We are sorry to tell you that it unquestionably rains a lot and surprisingly roughly evenly throughout the year. Our peninsula juts out into the sea/ocean and thus, being farthest west, we are the first of the British main island landmass to receive, the most commonly prevailing winds; named the 'westerly's. This, as most geography students know, means that the air rises as it hits land, and then it rains. (As water is deemed to be the new Gold, Cornwall may one day again be rich in another valued resource if storage space is created!)

Cornwall formally has what is known as a 'temperate maritime climate'. This means warm but not hot summers and cooler rather than cold winters. As an example we had a couple of days of snow when the Beasts from the East hit GB in 2018, but then the snow cleared and the day after that, you'd never have guessed it had snowed at all. It did repeat but the winter of 2019 certainly evidenced our counties warmth in comparison with the rest of GB. Equally, we find that the hot is really brief, and the mild and warm days are more common for the summer. The Cornish call a general mist and rainy drizzle 'mizzle,' this can be extensively persistent on the higher ground, such as the Moor and on the Cornish Alps near St Austell.

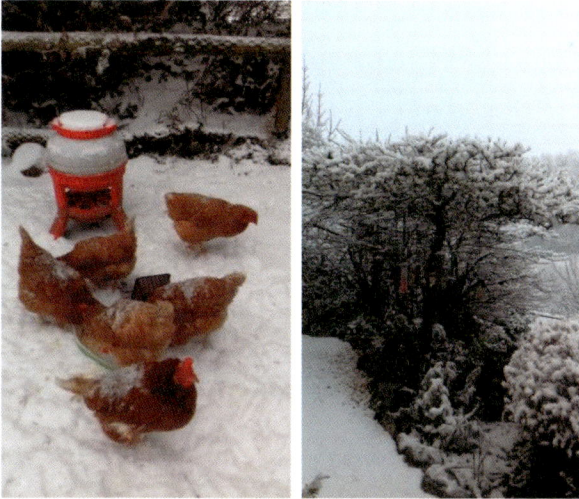

The evidence: The chickens handled it well considering they are battery rescues and had never walked before release let alone in snow!

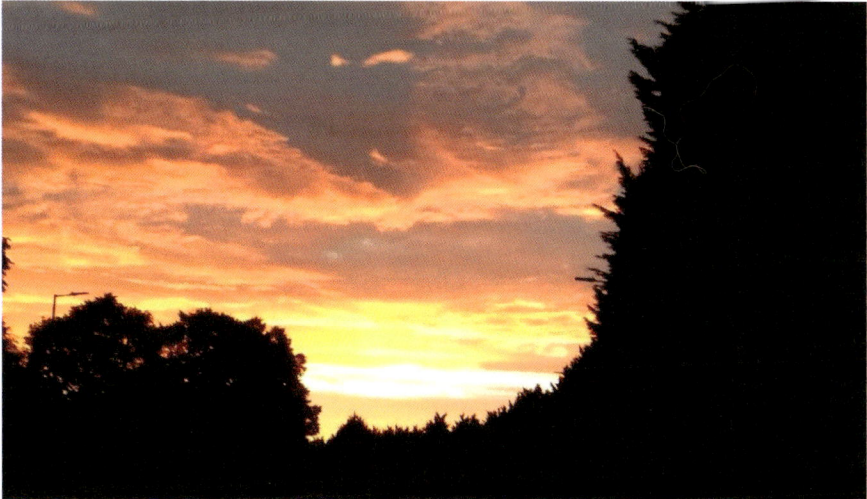

Sun setting in our Wild West.

During the National BBC summaries of rainfall and temperatures for the up'n coming dates, Cornwall has to take at closest Cardiff to ponder the next days' weather. Of course, if one watches the local news (Spotlight-other news reports for weather are available) you will get more localised weather patterns shared; this appears to demonstrate quite how we are literally out on a limb here. Cornwall did not get its' own weather station until 1978 when Camborne opened its' doors and started measuring the temperature, rainfall, and pressures.

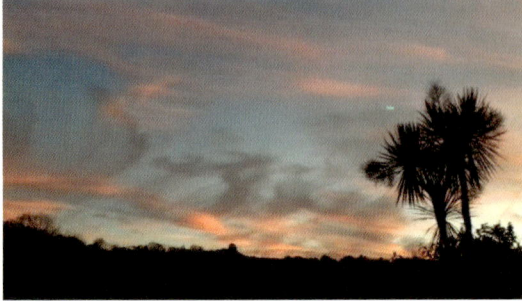

Red sky at night.......

Average temperatures obviously vary dependent on the *number* of years they are taken over, and *the year in* which taken, as well as *where* they are taken. Cornwall has numerous micro climates, but each can demonstrate all seasons in one day; to re-iterate a point; the weather changes remarkably quickly here. Also, it must be noted that the north and south coasts can have two very varying climate experiences at any one time; as a sea breeze in one direction blows it on to the land on one coast and off the often cliff-protected other.

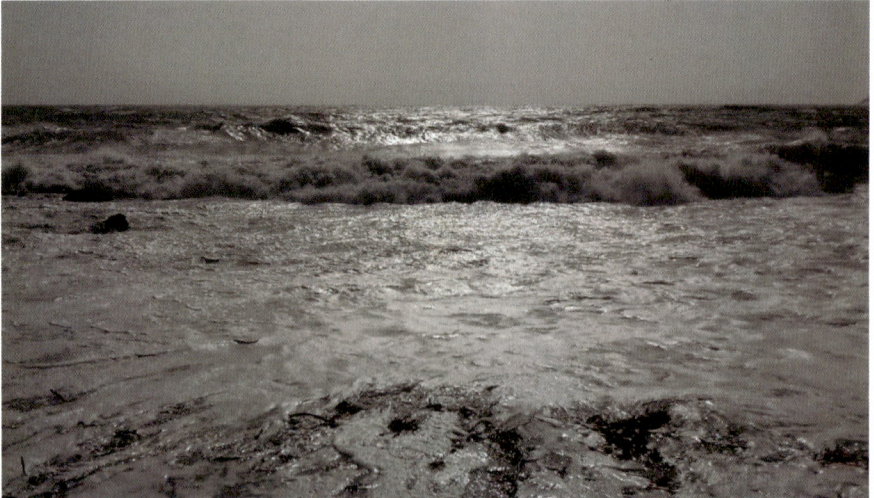

Some stats to ponder; remembering as Benjamin Disraeli said: "There are lies, damn lies and statistics", and as Mark Twain commented: "Facts are stubborn things, but statistics are pliable."

Temperatures.

	Jan	Feb	Mar	Apr	May	Jun	Jul	Aug	Sep	Oct	Nov	Dec
°C	6	6	7	8	11	14	16	16	15	12	9	8
°F	43	43	45	46	52	57	61	61	59	54	48	46

Rainfall.

	Jan	Feb	Mar	Apr	May	Jun	Jul	Aug	Sep	Oct	Nov	Dec
mm	110	90	100	60	60	70	60	60	70	110	100	120
Days	25	21	22	20	18	19	20	21	19	23	25	23

Hourly Sun per Day.

	Jan	Feb	Mar	Apr	May	Jun	Jul	Aug	Sep	Oct	Nov	Dec
Hours	2	3	4	6	7	7	7	7	5	4	3	2

Sea Temperatures.

	Jan	Feb	Mar	Apr	May	Jun	Jul	Aug	Sep	Oct	Nov	Dec
°C	10	9	9	10	11	13	16	17	16	14	12	11
°F	50	48	48	50	52	55	61	63	61	57	54	52

The Demographics (People stuff).

The advice given, often, is: to avoid both politics and religion especially at dinner parties; but some of us do so enjoy breaking that social convention! Therefore, as a pre-apology: please note that we have tried to put the following information in an objective and unbiased way, and we ask any forgiveness from those who choose to brave the following and engage in the subject if we veer towards the subjective.

Cornwall is one of 6 recognized Celtic nations; the others are: Scotland, Ireland, Wales, Brittany and the Isle of Man. The Kernow people's status was awarded the European Framework Convention for the Protection of National Minorities in 2014.

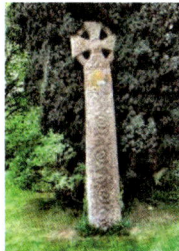

One of 200 stone Celtic crosses; marking the routes to sacred sites.

Firstly, the big political picture: The Conservatives have, in 2018 and 2019, control of Kernow and most of the West of Britain. Some find this unusual as there is much poverty (as we will see in a wee while). The closest answer Chrys has found in argument, debate and discussion on such matters is that Cornwall has not ever had a substantial Union representing the trades and services. Today, a high percentage of the workforce completes illegal numbers of hours and has no representation against possibly unjust and 'overexpecting' bosses. Conversely this can be seen as necessary to preserve businesses and thus still provide employment!

The Cornish have a strong local identity; the political party is called Mebyon Kernow, describing itself as a progressive left-of-centre party, 'striving to build a confident and outward-looking Cornwall and that (it) hopes for the power to take decisions directly affecting the people of Cornwall, locally'. Their policies are founded on three core values:

- Prosperity for all
- Social justice
- Environmental protection

The 2016 film 'Bad Education' was based in Cornwall and rather sarcastically, wethinks, raised awareness about the idea of the Cornish wish for liberation from the hands of Westminster. Additionally around the same time there was a fake news story about the 'Ooh Argh Ayy' burning Rick Stein's restaurant: it emerged to not have any validity at all, however amusing the joke about the IRA rhyme may be seen to be.

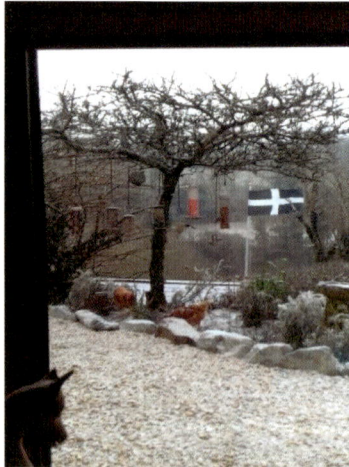

The Kernow flag flying on a colder Kernow day.

The flag is understood to be this design for two alternative reasons; either it was King Mark's flag during the Dark Ages or, more poetically St. Piran; The Patron Saint of mining and Kernow itself discovering tin as it shone white against the coals and blackened timbers in a fire.

Away from the slightly subjective now and on to the objective numbers..............

Cornwall's resident population in 2017 was 549,404 but the numbers are said to quadruple during the high season when the 'emmets' (see Chapter 8) arrive! There are 83 English counties excluding the Scillies (Population 2,280; 2017) and Greater London making Cornwall the 40th in population size.

Cornwall's population has been gradually rising. There was a 6.7% growth in population between the 2001 and 2011 census'. This number is 33,000 which is higher than any one Kernow town's populations sizes. The increase is primarily people over 40, with a decline in number for those under 39 and more importantly an accentuated decline of those aged 16-29. (The next census has not happened so information here is obviously somewhat dated).

Thank goodness this youth drain is slowing, seemingly because of an increase in Higher Education facilities and because more employment offers are becoming available. These general facts remain worrying when considering that; Britain's aging population is already showing signs of a troubling weight and pressure on the health and social care services. These services do not increase their staff number when the 'emmets' arrive. The strain is thus really heavy on the police, fire and health; their budgets and their even harder than normal working staff. Oops, gone a little off the objective again-this is difficult for us to avoid!!

Truro can be said to be a city since it has a Cathedral-it is beautiful, and worth a visit. St Austell our local town Historic Market town is the largest with a population of 27,400 but it has suburbs and outlying conurbations making the actual population closer to 34,700. It is very practical and functional but some would say not the prettiest. All Saint's Church is welcoming and beautiful but obviously not as large as the cathedral.

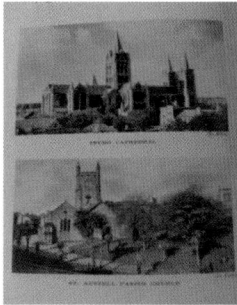

Image taken from Ward Lock's; South Cornwall, Ten Maps and Plans. The Fair Britain series.

Cornwall's population is 98.2% white-which troubles the writers frequently especially as Chrys who was reared in the extremely multi-ethnic and therefore multi-cultural West London. The sea of white faces can be disconcerting and unfamiliar to her and it can take a 'towny' some time to adjust to this pale populace. Ridiculously it can make one remark, internally, when there's a person of colour in Cornwall especially out of high season. The lack of multi-culturalism is often compared to 1950's Britain. If there is any prejudice in Cornwall let's stress it's generalised and aimed against anyone from across the Tamar and not to do with skin colour per se. (Especially the Devonians!)

About 60% of the Cornish population define themselves Christian, 30% declare no religious affiliation at all, 9% (ish) not declaring their religion. The largest minority religion was Buddhism at 0.32% of people reporting they were Buddhist, followed by Muslim (0.16%), Hindu (0.10%) and Jewish (0.07%). Again, this can feel unusual and limiting in perspective if one comes from a predominantly mixed cultural area but also interesting and 'oldy worldy'!

The language unsurprisingly is 98% English (as the first language) followed by Polish with only 464 people declaring Cornish their first language. (Again the above stats are from the 2011 census). FYI In 2019 a new TV station speaking Cornish has been launched.

The population of Cornwall, as said, is aging statistically with many Londoners (seemingly primarily those from the South West of London) and Midlanders, retiring and moving in search of the 'Good Life' in their final years. Chrys has a theory that people head the way the most convenient roads flow so the North East Londoners, for instance, head to Essex and Suffolk.

Anyway, back to the point of course we have the aforementioned standardised service industries here and much of the working age population is employed within them; police, schools, health and social care. The historical mining industries went in to decline when cheaper overseas imports invaded the market of tin, gold, silver and china clay. None the less St Austell's French-owned Imerys is still a large employer.

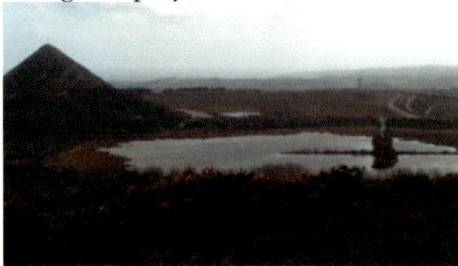

One of the pyramids created from the china clay industry's waste near St. Austell, part of an area named the Cornish Alps.

Much of the employment tends to be seasonal, namely in farming and tourism which can be irregular; another industry that again, provides no assured income is that of fishing. Therefore, unless one is an owner/manager or in a state provision or large company like Imerys, the populace commonly lives on zero hour contracts (if contractual at all) and minimum wages are more the norm. As previously noted, Unions barely exist in Cornwall and the less wealthy often work torturous hours to pay high prices. The tourist season prices do not go down once the 'emmets' leave so treats like theatre, cinema and restaurants can be unaffordable for many of the locals. Even though in some places at least, the car parking prices are reduced out of season. The best quote Chrys heard when doing a volunteering session at a local homeless hostel is: "The beauty disguises the poverty". OK rant over!

On a brighter note: Thank goodness for the fast Broadband's wide coverage that helps provide Cornish inhabitants with another often lucrative employment option!

Some background Cornish economic information for those that may be interested further. FYI this may be even more weighty than above but the umbrella perspective can help with the understanding, wethinks!.

Cornwall is one of the poorest areas in the United Kingdom with wages being 77.4% the UK average. Kernow has a GDP of £10.7 billion in 2016 which is 69% per cent of the European average. (GDP being the cash value of all goods and services). Cornwall is one of only four UK areas that qualify for these 'poverty-related' grants from the European Social Fund.

As one of the European Union's Objective One funding recipients, Kernow has qualifed as an area that meets the following criteria: to be an 'area where prosperity, measured in Gross Value Added per head of population is 75% or less of the European average'. Kernow has for many years fitted this bill. (GVA is another more complicated equation to judge the economic value created by goods and services in an area, but this time minus the costs of raw materials used)

So here we go; are you feeling brave? If not then move on to another subheading, otherwise hold tight to your seats and breathe deeply, as if plunging in to a cold sea...

This first book is being written in the year when no-one can avoid the 'B' word (Brexit, for those that have picked it up in a charity shop in the year 2050 and the 'B' word is not the current hot topic.) To clarify: it's when the British public were given an option to leave the European Union. Cornwall decidedly voted 'out' and interestingly perhaps, the Scillies voted to remain.

To expand on this point, Cornwall has received £1billion in aid over the past 15 years with more than £400 million assured until 2020 however there will expectedly be a shortfall if our National government does not subsidise the county!

On a positive note Kernow's GVA has increased by 4.1% whereas the current UK growth rate is in comparison 2.9%. To detract from the positive almost immediately; this is primarily due to the real estate sector-see below.

Cornwall's exports are second from the lowest (Cumbria) when compared to national exports.

This brings us on to the very sticky issue of second home ownership in Kernow. Many villages literally appear to die 'out of season', due to local shops, pubs, Post Offices and other necessary community services closing for lack of winter trade. Chrys; herself guilty of bringing town money to a rural location (and raising prices for the local potential buyers) was told by a North Coast estate agent that many villages are up to 70% second home owners.

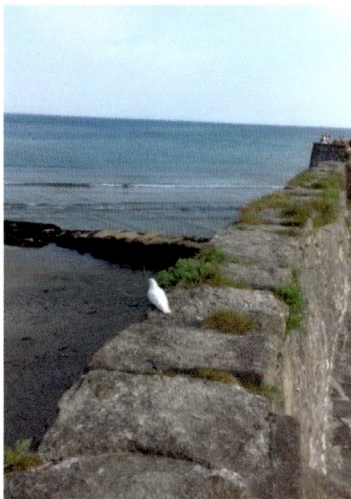

A Charlestown Dove looking out towards the mussel beds in St Austell Bay-to sooth whilst braving this section of the book!.

Cornwall's farmers and fishermen have also benefitted from the EU's Common Agricultural Policy and Common Fisheries Policy respectively. Cornwall generally has received tens of millions of pounds per year in structural and convergence funds to support local economic growth and communities. A good example of this is the park and ride service and development in Truro.

Some more stats for those brave and hardy reading souls who have ventured thus far; In September 2017 there were 235,859 people in employment. 174,959 of those were employees on average receiving £17,873 and 22% (52,266) were self-employed, whose income was £11,500 (both quoted as a median values). Part time employment provides for roughly one third of all workers, and there were 25,000 workless households. Those receiving Job Seekers Allowance is flexible with the seasons but is running in 2018 at around 3000 person.In a related earnings survey only Conwy in Wales and Moray in Scotland fared worse on wages.

Income, as said, is very seasonal for the tourist accommodation providers too but they do frequently get offered support from financial services with delayed mortgage payments and business rates. The private sector pay is lower across most sectors of employment.

Cornwall's council website; that few dare to broach has 2012 figures that show; only 2% of people are employed in agriculture, farming, fishing and mining. 6% in construction and property. 7% in the motor trade, transport and storage sector. Communications, information, finance, insurance, professional, scientific, technical, business and administration is at 12% Maybe we wouldn't be surprised to see that accommodation, food, arts, entertainment and recreation is at 20% there are 27% are employed in manufacturing, wholesale and retail! . Finally the largest sector is public services employing 28% of the working population.

Many companies actually pay less in Cornwall than elsewhere in the country for the same job; the formula used to assess paid wages appears to ignore the expense of living in the area and takes house prices as a factor.

A real time example; working for supply teaching agencies at a secondary level pays £135-£150/ day in North Lincolnshire and is £105/day in Cornwall. Primary supply teachers wages go down from £110 to £85.90/ day with the same areas comparison. To perhaps over accentuate the point; in addition to lower wages Cornwall also has some of the highest costs of living in the UK.

Housing costs are some of the most expensive outside of the South East and London, with price to earnings ratios in popular locations often exceeding 10 times. This is, we guess, to be expected when one considers the influx population and its spending potential. House prices (UK average, early 2018 was £224,144 and Cornwall's average was £274,350) with above average levels of unemployment. So take a gasp of relief if you braved the section above as if plunged in to the Cold Sea and having the Cold Water Immersions flight and fight reaction, then rest, digest and heal with brighter and lighter information.

Crime

As could perhaps be expected, Cornwall rates fairly well in terms of crime figures. Car theft is generally around a tenth of the national average, as is robbery, with burglaries running at roughly half the UK rate. The blip is theft from cars, with nearly double the national average in some areas of Cornwall – this being a crime that is often associated with tourist regions.

The Arts, Entertainment and 'things to do' including some food info

Chrys likes to joke that one comes to Cornwall, pretentiously, to paint or write primarily influenced by the light as well as the 'dreckly' mode of being. (See Chapter 8) The fact is that many, many of the Cornish folk do have a most amazing creativity, maybe due to an almost old fashioned way of creative thinking with interesting language skills, or is it due to the inspiring land and seascapes?

It can also be noted that often where folk have struggled and faced a lot of adversity, literally in the face of life and death, creativity can be increased. In rural and seagoing areas the life of people, fish and animals tend to be more at risk, and death more visible. This 'face to faceness' with elemental extremes, without the towns' sanitizing effects can be seen to create deeper existential thinking (Oh, are we back to Sartre?). In summary; one has to ponder life and existence more deeply in the face of death.

So, as not to appear overdramatic, in this section regarding the dramas of life and, again to suggest some of you may wish to journey along this brief and small diversionary tangent and some may wish to forgo...

It can be noted that societies that function well and fully, where the populace are judged to be 'happy', tend to produce less passionate and deep literature or theatre. Inequalities and recognized social injustices can be seen to create a fighting spirit, where one wants to challenge the status quo. The arts are often the chosen channel to do this. Kernow has prolific localised plays and performances that challenge difficulties 'head on' both politically and artistically.

Therefore or not, encased in a landscape of inspiring and motivating views and dramatic nature, Cornwall creates fabulous ventures and is a leading cultural mover, with influences on the world stage. Consider the environmental teachings of The Eden Project and its model being applied in the far off foreign lands such as China, and the spectacularly creative and originally styled theatrical dramas of the Kneehigh and Miracle Theatre Companies to name only a couple of our current favourites.

Historically, this narrow shire full of mystery and history has of course helped to inspire writers such as Daphne Du Maurier and more recently Rosamunde Pilcher. The list is forever growing and creativity is rife in all styles of creative presentation. It's difficult to visit an area in Cornwall and to return home without a beautiful painting or perhaps a sculpture by a talented local artist. Or maybe to bring home memories of a play seen, perhaps beautifully performed at The Minnack or recalling the experience one has had strolling dreckly around the New Tate at St. Ives.

One cannot ignore the BBCs Poldark series which has been spectacularly well received and sometimes obsessively watched. Aiden Turner, the main actor has turned a few heads and has even had fans, often women of 'our certain age' traipsing around the county hoping for a glimpse. A friend of Chrys's has this urge and speaks of the Canadian and American women she has met all held back by security staff when watching the filming of Poldark!

On a smaller and very local scale every New Year has numerous village pantos being performed. The Cornish enjoy the delights of fancy dress more than elsewhere in the country, especially notable with the Cornish Carnivals. New Year's Eves in the pubs demonstrates some fabulous examples of the dressing up games to be witnessed or participated in. Smaller theatre productions and interesting speakers are common in the towns, for instance at The St Austell Arts Centre. London's West End's theatre productions commonly perform at The Hall for Cornwall (Truro; FYI shut for refurbishment from June 2018 for 2 years)

Cornwall holds tight to many traditions, brass bands living on as heritage from the mining era. Concerts and band practices are clear signs of how much past time are still celebrated here; BBC Radio Cornwall has a programme of Brass Band Music on a Sunday afternoon. Dare we say another example of Kernow appearing like 1950s Britain?

Choirs are a very popular social affair in Kernow. The joys of hearing an outdoor (indoor renditions are also available) chorus of voices singing traditional tunes, keeping them well and truly alive for the future is a wonder to be experienced. Chrys especially enjoys 'Little Eyes' and the Kernow anthem 'Trelawny'; describing when 20,000 Cornish men marched on London!

The many fabulous pubs have regular open mike and local band music nights. Frequently the most marvellous of foods-the vegan options are increasing although only a few actual vegan restaurants currently exist; it is though rare to not have any choices. FYI and as a recommendation The Cornish Vegan in Truro won a Gold Award from the Cornish Tourism Board 2018/19

The 'carnists' amongst yourselves will be pleased to know the local animal products are seen as some of the best on the planet. The weather section shows how plentifully fed the grasses are for the grazing sheep and bovines, and the cleaner sea and ocean waters have prolific produce. We are also the only GB County with no factory farming! We are especially proud of this fact and hope 'long may it last'! The fishermen will be happier once the EU quotas are changed and thus sea food may be in even more abundance from local sources.

Cornwall is of course dotted with beautiful gardens and manor houses which include much traditional fine art as one would expect but Kernow, also offers the delight of gardens with extremely creative and alternative arts incorporated; for example Tremenheere sculpture garden over looking Penzance.(ATL)

We must not leave out the extensive alternative water sports that take place all around the coast, Chrys's favourite aside from the Wild Swimming is 'coasteering'; what excitement! There are converted quarries for inland water sports and other adventures to be had at sites such as Adrenalin Quarry (add to your list?). The North Coast is of course renowned for surfing and hosts the internationally renowned Boardmasters every year. Sailing, kayaking, water skiing, donuts etc. are all available during the high season and these may interfere with a Wild Swim be wise and check the events calendar!

Parking

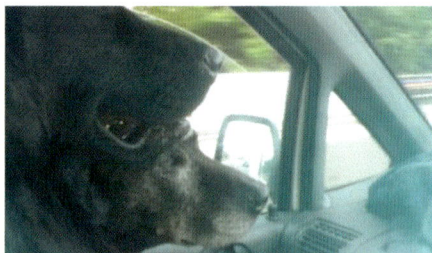

Do not leave dogs in cars please.

Most of the year round one can find a parking space near where one wants to visit-usually you have to pay even if with a Disability Blue Badge (you usually get one extra hour with it). BUT during the high season we would suggest to do, as the archetypal Germans are renowned to do; get there early and reserve your spot. A quick anecdote from a friend who tried to leave St Ives where they had accommodation parking after trying 3 other beach spots: Perrenporth, St Agnes and Newquay. The car full of hot and frustrated moods then had to journey around and go back to the hotel; as Cornwall was 'FULL' and there was nowhere to park. So be early or be late or out of season to guarantee a space, and be careful with your carfuls. Alternatively one can of course choose to the more environmentally friendly alternative and jump on the maximised public transport during high season.

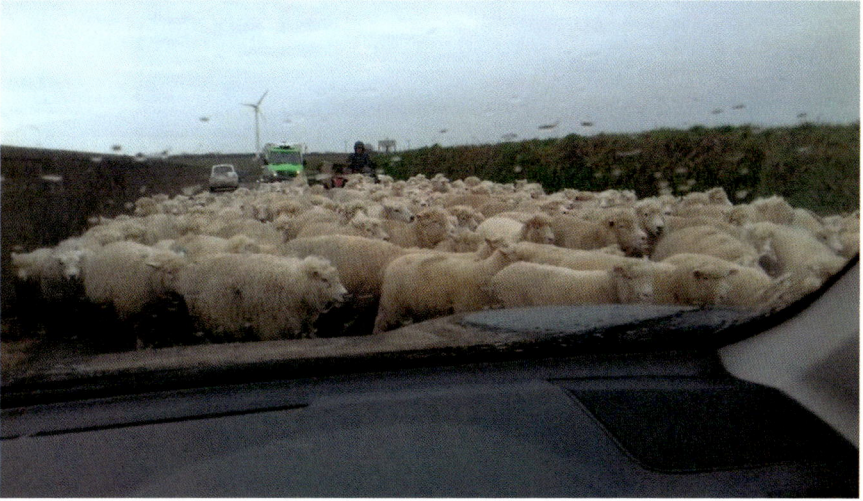

You may be forced to park where you may not have chosen too.

It may be worth having National Trust Membership as this means free parking at their sites except with a junior membership, thus a parking perk on top of exquisite views and places of interest. But of course this does not guarantee a space either.

As a useful tip-there are many slopes from the ridiculously steep to the gentle incline in Kernow, so we really recommend leaving your car in gear (unless automatic) when parked, and not leaving all the strain on the handbrake.

Whilst mentioning parking just a wee word about driving: Cornish hedges are often not as they seem. They are made of stone, thus an unwary driver may pull in to kindly let another pass on the considerably tight roads and damage their car. So please be careful. Cornish hedges are very much a visible presence within your Kernow experience and are a delight of wild flowers seasonally but as noted can be dangerous to the uninformed driver. Whilst we are on the subject of separation of one area from another please do look out for the fabulous Cornish stiles that dot the county; the great granite cornices are a marvellous site or seat when climbed on and over.

Ok so now we head to the first specific Wild Swim sites and hope you are now sufficiently suffused with multitudinous Kernow knowledge.

3. Goldiggins Quarry near the Hurlers, Bodmin Moor.

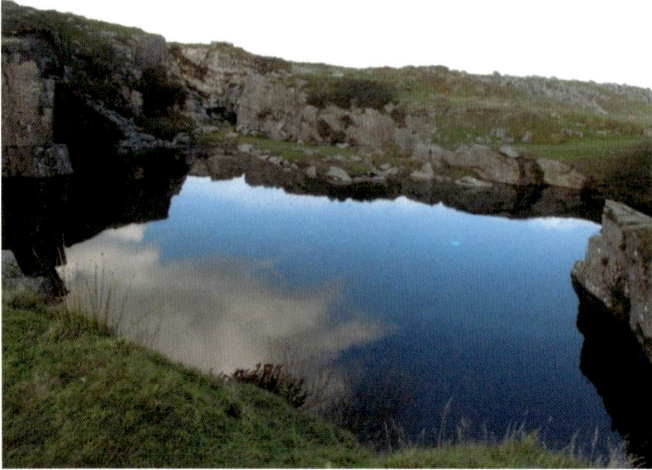

Bodmin appears to be a derivative of the shortened version and combination of Bod (later Bos) meaning dwelling place and 'menegh' meaning monks, therefore; the 'dwelling place of the monks'.

Minions Village has a FREE car park and our first sojourn is to the popular site for Wild Swimming close by at Goldiggins Quarry. Lying high on a jutting vertebra of Cornwall's granite spine on the frequently windswept, literally and metaphorically, outstanding Bodmin Moor. Easiest access to this absolutely beautiful wild historically, geologically and spiritually fascinating place is from the south east; closer to the town of Liskeard than to Bodmin Town itself.

Chrys had the entertaining experience of meeting a group of naturists who had intended crossing the moor 'au naturel'; the weather meant they were clad in clothes at the beginning of our chats. Once the hardy swimmers started dunking there was a variety added to the views within the landscape; there was an awful lot of flesh dangling from the 'certain aged' courageous homo sapiens!

The Minions is weenie and the highest village in Cornwall. and a delight to visit with a pub and two cafés for treats after the swim and walk.

Don't miss their Heritage Museum for deeper and wider Kernow knowledge. This is within the recently restored Houseman's Engine House where one can explore a permanent exhibition on the history and nature of the surrounding areas the mining past. The area surrounding Minions still clearly demonstrates evidence of the region's links with the historical Cornish mining tradition Redundant engine houses standing proud, and erect as a reminder of the tin and copper mining that took place here until early in the last century, when the last shaft named; the Prince of Wales (well we are in the Duchy) shaft closed around 1914. Many of the pump houses and spoil tips can still be seen.

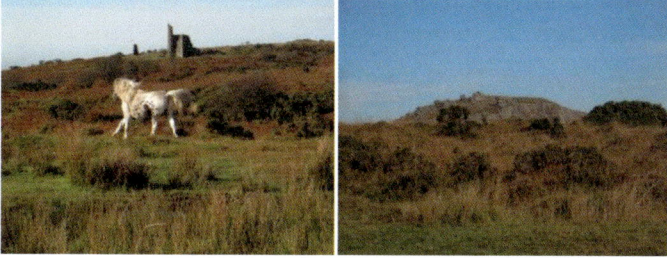

Most other villages and towns in Cornwall developed around an individual industry, but Minions grew to provide homes and resources for those who worked in railways, as well as quarrying and mining. Goldiggins mine, where we swam, and hope you will, was part of the Caradon Mining District. The railway at the Cheesewring opened in 1844 and was used to transport the silver-grey granite to Liskeard and Looe for export; the old track is still visible in parts, and is often used ramblers (clothed or not!) and by people riding tamed horses to explore and enjoy the area.

The surrounding area is thus swamped, and swampy, with fascinating places to explore. One of these is the 3 amazing standing stone circles named; the Hurlers. The story goes that the locals were playing Hurlers (a local game) on a Sunday. They were consequentially deemed to be punished for sacrilegious behaviour by being turned to stone. The truth of the matter is that the stones are spiritual and astronomical Bronze Age circles most likely carved and planted in to the ground about 1500 BC.

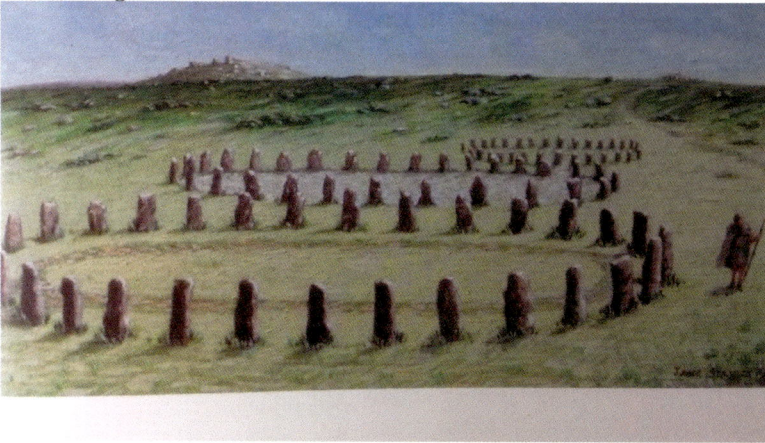

From a Brush with the Past; with thanks to Jane Stanley. The Hurlers with the Cheesewring on the horizon.

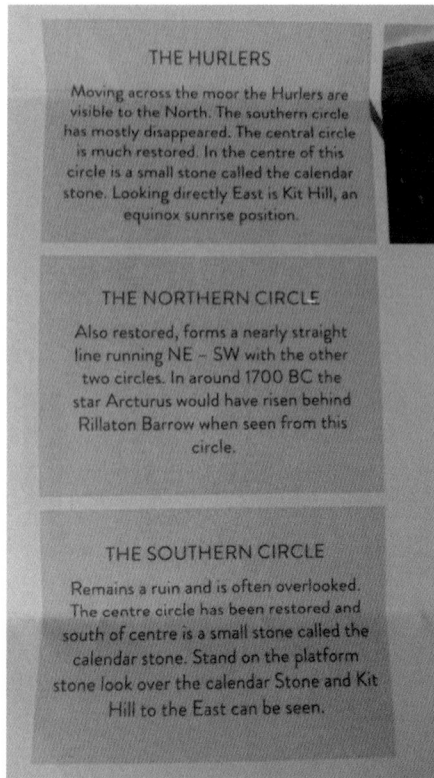

THE HURLERS

Moving across the moor the Hurlers are visible to the North. The southern circle has mostly disappeared. The central circle is much restored. In the centre of this circle is a small stone called the calendar stone. Looking directly East is Kit Hill, an equinox sunrise position.

THE NORTHERN CIRCLE

Also restored, forms a nearly straight line running NE – SW with the other two circles. In around 1700 BC the star Arcturus would have risen behind Rillaton Barrow when seen from this circle.

THE SOUTHERN CIRCLE

Remains a ruin and is often overlooked. The centre circle has been restored and south of centre is a small stone called the calendar stone. Stand on the platform stone look over the calendar Stone and Kit Hill to the East can be seen.

The Hurlers attracts visitors from all over the world who may also come to "Dowse" the stone circles and feel the energy that is said to come from them. Chrys was cynical at a sound testing equinox event, led by the Cornish Astronomical Society.(ATL) When attempting dowsing, she was rather interested to learn how the St Michaels' ley line crosses there running from St Michaels' Mount near Penzance through the Hurlers, on to Glastonbury tor on and on via many St Michael's Churches hitting the sea near Great Yarmouth.

The singing and chanting was said to extend the width and the intensity of the ley line energy; to later shrink when the sounds and volume quietened. Chrys used the dowsing rods and they undoubtedly swung around vigorously on their own. We highly recommend trying this. There is a lot of water there in pools; dowsing is often used to search for water, the rods can also be used to look for anything one attunes oneself to find! A Cornish friend tells tales of discovering lost cattle and stolen goods when attuning himself to their energies via dowsing rods! ATL of possible To Dos; a couple of old metal clothes hangers bent to right angles should suffice.

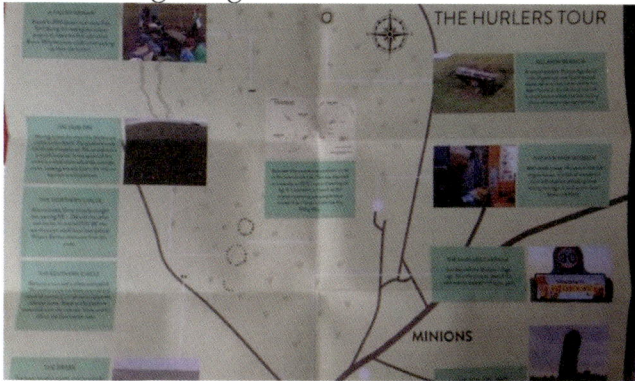

From 'Bright Stars: Dark Skies'. The Hurlers. A Self Guide Tour. This may be useful as well as adding an additional angle of interest. Many thanks.

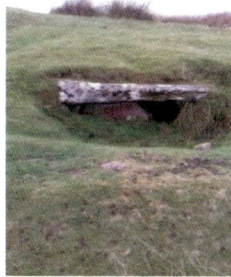

Close by, some 200 metres from the Hurlers to the north cast, is situated an Early Bronze Age burial chamber, it is 30 metres in diameter and once contained the remains of a human skeleton; beads; a spear head; pottery and the 'Rillaton' Gold Cup. The ribbed cup is small 80 millimeters in height and is believed to have originated in the Middle Ages The suggestions being that was it was brought to Cornwall by a trade route, or fashioned by local craftsmen who had seen similar products and copied the design. The original cup spent some time in the Royal families' household but now resides in the British Museum. All other artifacts from the sight have sadly been lost. A copy of the Rillaton Cup is now kept in the Cornwall Museum, Truro.

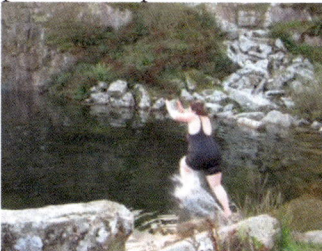

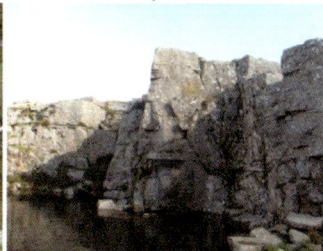

The Cheesewring stands in stark silhouette about 1.5 kilometres north across the moor. It is another fascinating aspect of this particular Wild Swimming

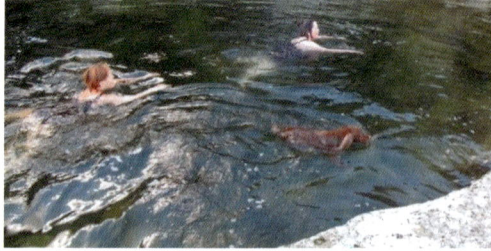

place to visit. The distinctive shape can be seen from most parts of the Minions moor. The shape has been the subject of many a debate, but we are now clear it is the result of weather erosion on the granite strata of the moor over many millennia.

Goldiggins Quarry was so named as Gold was found there in 1837 whilst the mine was being quarried for the more expected copper, tin and arsenic, all of which can be created within granite. We may recognise what gold, tin and copper metals can be used for, but we were unsure of the use of the metalloid arsenic as we only thought of it as a poison. So here's some more, future pub quiz, information; arsenic is poisonous in larger quantities, but is actually an essential dietary trace element needed in many species such as chicken; rat; goat; hamster and human! Arsenic and compounds of it are additionally used in the production of pesticides; treated wood products; herbicides and insecticides-although these applications are currently declining. Humans have also discovered its' use as a semi-conductor of electricity, thus use it in the making of technical devices.

This was our highest swim, we hope these pictures demonstrate the delight and joy of the sensations, the play and feel good factor involved.

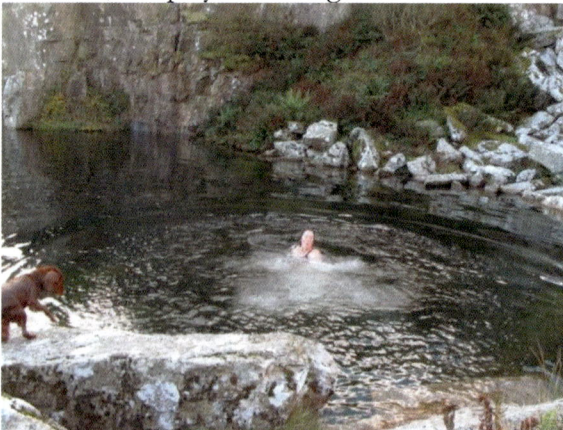

Dipping in to the Duchy

This 19th century spring fed quarry lake, sheltered by an amphitheatre of rock, can be remarkably much colder than the sea or river swims we include in this book. Cold static water can by physical laws, be much colder than flowing water. Thus we recommend all our previous health and safety advice be considered and (or) re-read just to be sure. For this particular swim there is a 15-30 minute walk depending on how many times one stops to look at the incredible views. If not shrouded in 'mizzle' one can see into Devon on an especially clear day. One could also stop to watch the wild ponies and local cattle meandering and wandering their territory. The heavy rainfall and the underlying granite are the cause of this area having poor drainage resulting in it being best used for 'livestock' grazing. Add to this image of 'faunic' delights, and 'faunic' gallivanting; wild horses and ponies, and you have it, a dream complete.

BEWARE of the fabled and mystical phantom panther like cat renowned as the Beast of Bodmin! This rural myth has in 2019 revived it self as rumours of giant black cats taking sheep and scaring wary walkers are again abound!

Less enticing, we think, as a story to describe where the Bodmin big beastie came from also sadly more likely version; is that the animal trainer Mary Chipperfield released three pumas into the wild following the closure of her Plymouth zoo in 1978.

An official investigation was carried out in 1995 and no evidence was found. BUT a large cat's skull was discovered not long after that conclusion was made, in the River Fowey by a boy. This was later said by the Natural History Museum to be a young male leopard. (Later shown to have been imported!) So there is 'rumour abound' but evidence proves not so thrilling as the dramatic tale/tail☺

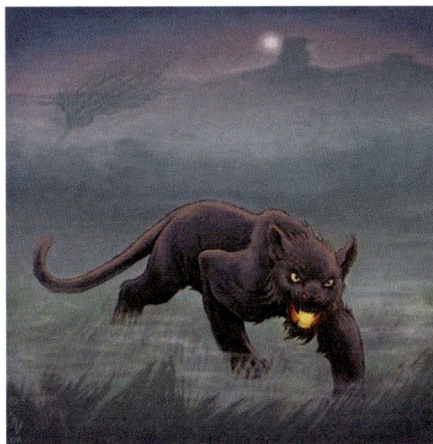

You have been warned!

4. Lostwithiel; River Fowey Swim.

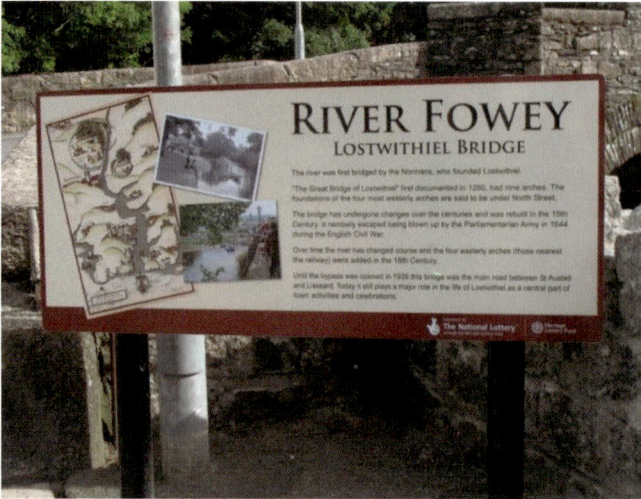

The name Lostwithiel is derived from the Cornish 'lostwydhyel,' meaning 'tail of a wooded area'.

This next venture of ours, and hopefully yours is a river swim just where the sea tides meet the land's runoff. To guarantee the deepest waters and avoid simply finding deepened pools to dunk in. As well as to avoid simply paddling for most of the time, one must first check if the sea is in. Tide times are available on many websites and little booklets at a lot of retail outlets. (See 'The When' in Chapter 1).

We went in for our Wild Water Swim by the historical Lostwithiel Bridge started in the mid 15th Century!

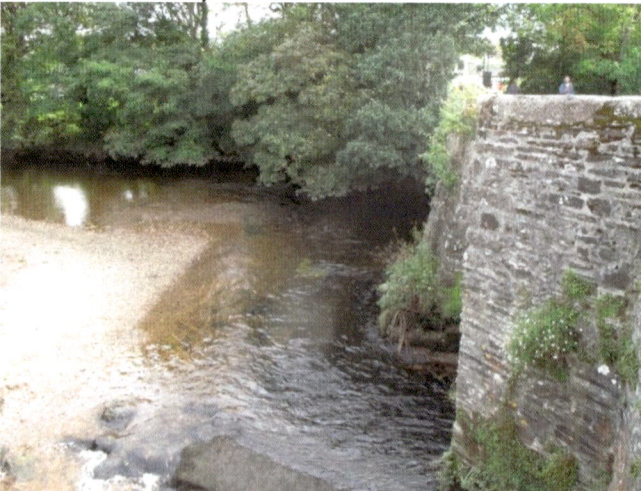

This is the River Fowey pronounced 'foye', which drains from its 177.5 km river basin that covers an area across south and central Bodmin Moor. (Please take note of the literal and alluvial connection of our swimming route!) With a river swim one must also ponder and consider recent rainfall as this will, somewhat obviously, affect the extent of the outward flows' speed, as well as the water mass. The Fowey water flows from a height of 290m on the moor, flowing down a length of 9km to Fowey-the 'well worth a visit' town at the estuary/sea. One can seasonally and on all winds except extreme easterlies take the Fowey to n fro Mevagissey Ferry(ATL)

The river runs through igneous granite; The Rock of Ages. As a reminder, or if you missed out the Geology in Chapter 2 we'll now briefly summarize; Igneous rock is formed from molten magma at extremely high temperatures, creating randomly interlocking crystals. The size depends very much on the rate of cooling-larger crystals have cooled more slowly and vice versa.

The river goes on to flow through Devonian slate-oh the 'arch enemies' from across the Tamar named again!-this was formed during the geological era named Devonian-funny enough. This slate was also created during South West England's mountain building era when the massive tectonic plates were colliding to form Pangea. As the continents eroded creating sand and mud sediment, which was consequently buried deeply, over time immemorial and under weight and heat it eventually turned to rock.

Delights that can appear with these formations are fossils. Fish fossils can be found from the ancient deltas and lagoons around Lostwithiel; worth an explore, wethinks. Further towards the sea, there are mudstones called Straddon Grits and Meadon beds; which also date from the Devonian period.

Historically, there was copper and china clay mining in the area, and to make you aware, and therefore beware; nearby there were also cyanide and the element titanium mines- extreme ends of the danger spectrum. Cyanide being rather reactive and the tough metal being very much less so. Therefore, the river waters can be 'sedimentally' contaminated with metalferrious compounds although the mines are now derelict, there is still a risk of runoff. We remain seemingly unaffected by any of these possible contaminants, thankfully.

Cyanide also has alternative uses to poisoning like arsenic. Cyanide, we think sadly, is used in the processing of acrylic materials-the Marine Strandings Network reported research about the consequences of the small plastic fibres entering the marine food chains at their conference 2019. It's also used in the production of other plastics, grrrr, as well as such actions as electroplating and supporting the hardening of iron and steel. It can interestingly be found in the pits of cherries and the seeds of apples. Chrys has heard that eating the apple pips with the flesh is one of the reasons our closest primate relatives have such far fewer cancers! So it can be good. Titanium was discovered in Cornwall and is renowned for its non-reactivity and it's strength to density ratio. Many of us Homo sapiens are bionically re-made using this element for spinal rods and more.

Rivers can also contain the runoff from agricultural exploits, thus pesticides and other biochemicals can be in the water. Not trying to put you off, but maybe wiser not to dunk your head too deeply and never drink the water (if it can be avoided).

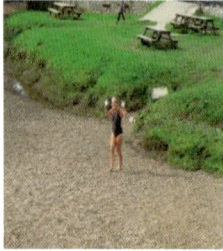

Currently near Lostwithiel there is heathland, moorland and rough pasture. The upper reaches are broadleaf coniferous and mixed plantation woodland. The mid to lower sections are rural and, maybe to over-accentuate the point, mean that the water can be contaminated with farm waste after extreme rainfall. Landscapes close by are recognized as both Areas of Great Scientific and also of having Historical Value therefore we suggest going walkabout!

The river was once much deeper and wider for the export ships to take the tin to Europe. At one point Lostwithiel was the second largest port in the south of England but the river silted up with the deposition of waste from the moor's mines.

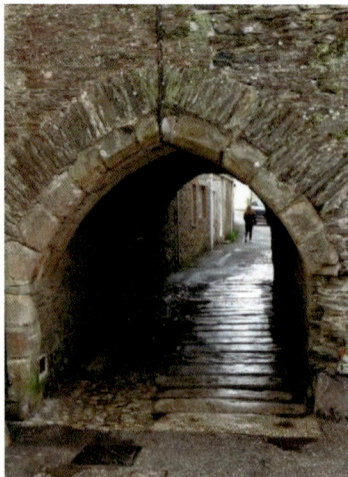

The town was founded around 1200 AD by the Normans to export tin being Kernow's capital during the thirteenth century. Lostwithiel later became the most important 'stannary' town in Kernow; a 'stannary' town was the administrative centre for a region. The town's principle purpose was to collect the 'tin coinage' to pay it on to the Duchy of Cornwall. This contravened the Magna Carta never-the-less it was not abolished until 1838. The tinners had enormous power Stannary Law could over ride Common Law and thus people were able to ignore some of the laws of the land! Another aspect of why Cornwall has become the Wild West; wethinks..

The town may have lost its political and financial prowess and has become instead renowned for its artistic, social and community gatherings such as its fabulous festivalsfor example; LostFest, a week-long carnival in the summer; arts and crafts festival; a beer festival; food and cider festivals in the October, as well as a Dickensian evening in December.

Lostwithiel has a lovely selection of antique shops and other retail delights. The library contains a great collection of books on Cornwall. As is common place in Kernow, there are fabulous hotels, restaurants and pubs to explore along the quaint streets. So make more of a day of it post Wild Swim, perchance visiting the close by Restormal Castle to take in the history and the striking views to get the true 'lie of the land' or maybe use the town as a base to extend your travels and Swims!

We parked at the stations, payed and displayed, ready for a dunk much to the amusement of several commuters and shoppers. One must be hardy and resilient to social judgement and possible ridicule as well as hardy and resilient to temperatures when venturing a Wild Swim. One must maybe reflect on Sartre again (Chapter 1) and fundamentally create your own identity whatever others think. Possibly again a factor in the 'certain age' of the women involved in creating this book! The now familiar and prolific reactions demonstrated by these commuters and general onlookers had become common place to us. Comments and looks inferring; 'we must be mad,' were clearly projected across to us as they (dare we say; the less adventurous homo sapiens) passed us by, being fully dressed, in fact winter attired, as we adventured forth with towels, flip flops and cossies. One does so hope that deep down they may had some respect and admiration at least for our courage? Meanwhile the canines seemed to show a wish to join us. Be more dog.

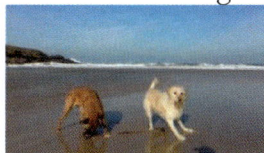

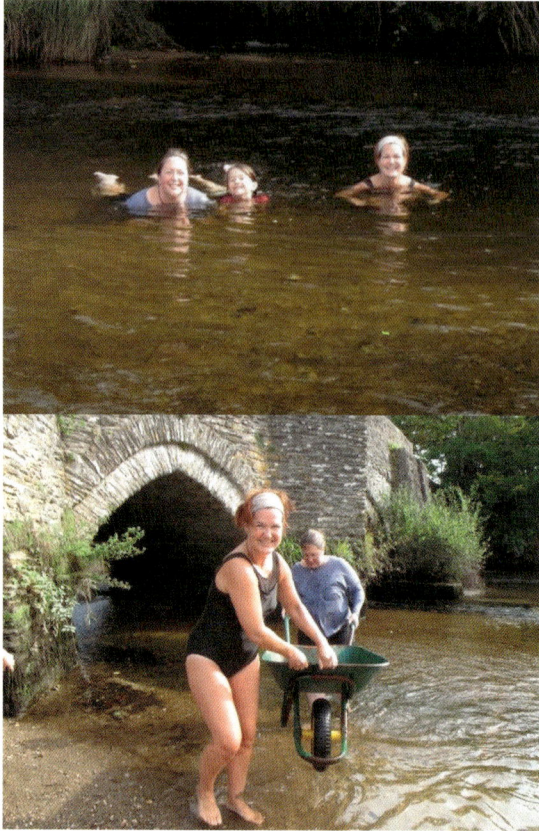

We did our social duty as per usual by helping tidy the left behind, or washed down litter from the area, as we highly recommend and overtly nag that you do the same wherever you go. We then enjoyed this swim as a real alternative Wild Swim. We of course had a little play about too.

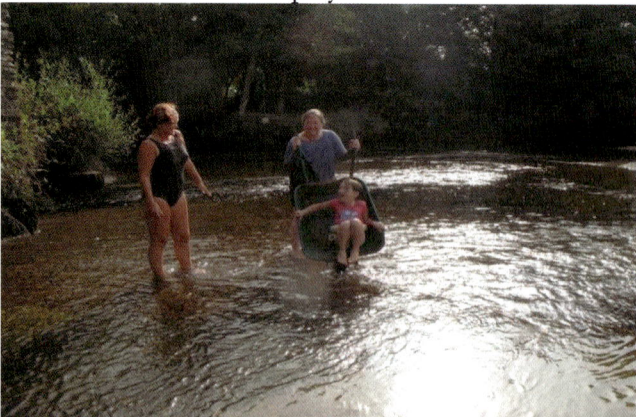

5. St Austell and Mevagissey Bay area. Otherwise known as the Cornish Riviera; All the Ps; Polkerris, Porthpean, Pentewan, and Portmellon. With mention of Gorran Haven, Mevagissey, Charlestown, Menabilly, Fowey and Trenarren.

Most of the above entitled Wild Swimming sites will only truly appear 'Wild' out-of-season but all lie within a recognised Area of Outstanding Beauty. FYI One third of Cornwall has this status! These Bays are therefore popular tourist areas and the sea will be much warmer during the high season; so if a real novice to outdoor swimming then perchance choose these times and places? The beaches will be covered with and the sea filled with 'emmets'. Tame warm busy water is, of course lovely and very acceptable!

This chapter flows in order from east to west across and along the Bays.

Polkerris.

In Cornish; Pollkerys, meaning fortified pool but one would struggle to find pool other than the harbour's safe protected waters.

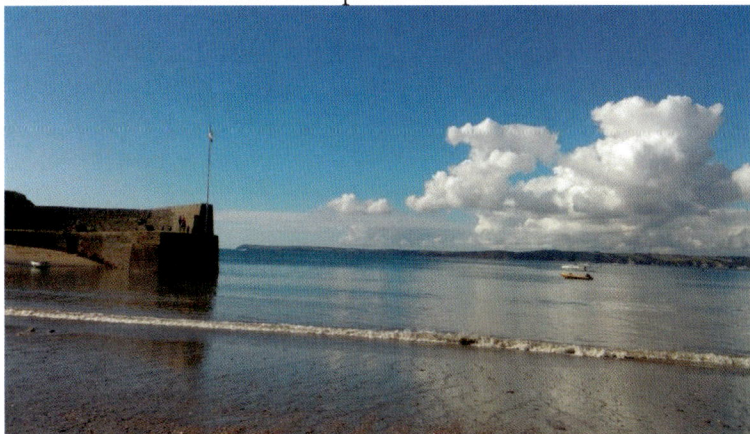

Polkerris is delightfully sheltered and protected by the harbour wall. The beach is the final point of the steep sloping, exquisitely quaint and tiny hamlet. The Rashleigh Pub and Sam's Diner are the guardians to the beaches' entrance, this area being part of the Rashleigh family estate.

It is best to park in the pay and display car park and walk the 2/3 minutes downhill through the hamlet usually and possibly obviously more on the tired uphill climb! The pub car park is small and tight but if out of season or if one is definitely either; cleaning the beach and/or eating and drinking there, then this is of course a viable free option.

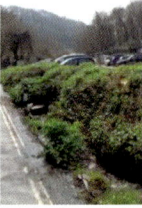

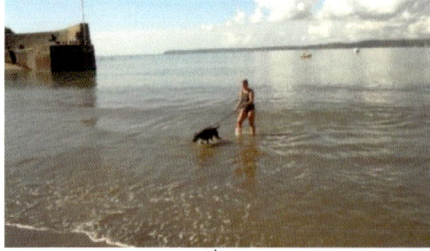

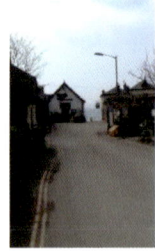

Polkerris was known from the 16th Century for its pilchard (Sardina pilchardus) fishing. Seining was used (see below in Portmellon section concerning Gorran Haven). The dark, and somewhat menacing, domineering massive and very structurally sound and thus 'walkable' harbour wall was built in 1775.

The seining company that built it didn't survive its centenary and closed in 1870. The entire beach, its water sports business and cafe were sold in 2016, with an 8 year lease for around £250,000. Due to the high, and clearly difficult to estimate, number of 40,000 visitors per year; we highly recommend swimming here out of season as the waters get full of crafts; from paddle boards to visiting yachts and dinghies.

The beach is small even at low tide but has a boat load of character. Sam's was the old Lifeboat housing which was built in 1859 for £138 4S and was in use in St Austell Bay, until the lifeboat service went to Fowey in 1922. Chrys is a regular visitor here and has never found the beach, thus far, with an extreme angle of slope into the water, therefore Polkerris may be a good introduction to a Wild Swim but please consider and include the above advice about water crafts

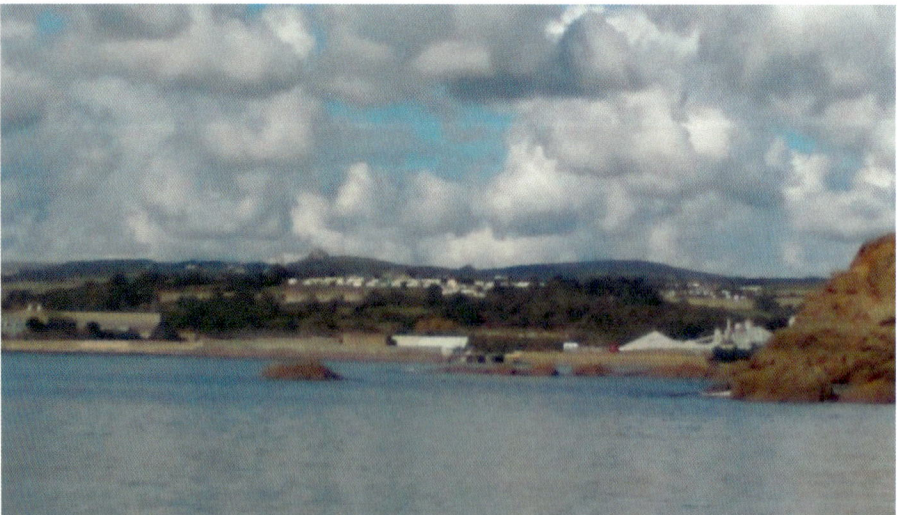

Polkerris overlooks Par with its' China Clay Industrial buildings and if one climbs over the headland towards the east you reach Menabilly and Polridmouth Cove Bay. Menabilly is overlooked by Kilmarth, the long term, and last home of the famous Cornish writer Daphne du Maurier. This is where she wrote 'The House on the Strand' and 'Rebecca'. 'Rebecca' is often viewed as her most famous piece of work; this is believed to be written with the property on the beach at Menabilly in mind, with the area additionally inspiring other later works. Du Maurier obviously fell in love with the Lodge on the beach, living and rearing her children near there for 20 years. Dogs are welcome all year around at Polridmouth Cove Bay but only out of season at Polkerris.

One can follow the South West Coast further east from here back to Fowey. This journey is across wide open sloping fields of grass or heading west one can venture to the Gribben Lighthouse. So much to see and do!

Porthpean.

Porthpean means 'little cove' and is yet another exquisite village close to the town of St Austell. It is split between Higher and Lower Porthpean. It is worth being dropped off at the top on the higher road from Pentewan to St Austell and traversing through the households to the sea, or again by walking the South West Coastal path to this beauty. One walks down, and down, and if via the roads, one can really relish the views and delights along the way. The church is quaint and picturesque, seating only 48. Visitors are made very welcome when attending services to have a sing-along and/or a prayer (or ten; if need be!). The parking close to the beach is now pay and display all year round.

If the tide is in there's not a whole lot of beach, but when out it's small but welcoming with the additional fun of rock climbing around both sides. If one goes left-looking out to sea there are interesting holes in the rocks and rocks that jut out to sea where one can jump or dive from and then swim back as well as a 'man sized', 'man made' cave to discover. Seasonally the Porthpean Beach shop and cafe, water sports centre and public toilets open.

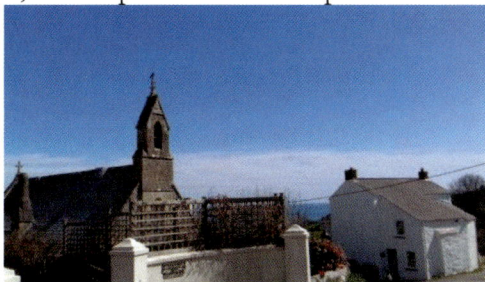

Porthpean has a single hull sailing club thus it's probably best to avoid Sundays and possibly Wednesday evenings from the Spring to Autumn if you want to Wild Swim Kernow here.

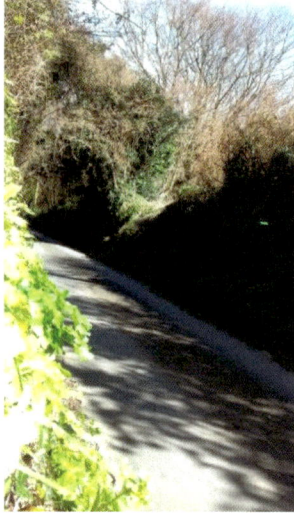

The walk down from the West end is a 'helluva' lot steeper than the picture shows!

Chrys watched and met a most courageous swimmer there last year. There were many fully wet suited swimmers about 150 metres out to sea for what seemed ages longer than Katherine and Chrys ever swam together. Amongst them a man, only in his trunks, who on returning to the beach was questioned about his hardiness by Chrys. He helpfully, wethinks, said how they were all local runners adding to their training. He explained how he had managed to acclimatize so competently, by being immersed in the cold water every day, extending the length of time doing so! A great plan if one is dedicated or able enough.

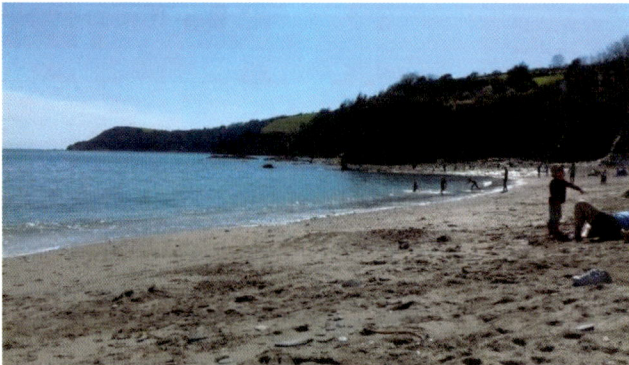

Porthpean beach looking west towards Blackhead and Trennaren.

A Cornish maid describes the tourism being so rife in the 1950s that a bus would to n fro to Porthpean beach from St Austell town every half an hour during the high season! This is no longer available, but again it is on the SW Coastal Path as well as only a little jut of land away from Charlestown. Charlestown is where many besotted people are currently visiting, hoping to catch a glimpse of Aiden Turner or to see where some of the scenes from (the more recent) Poldark were filmed. Poldark is a BBC TV series made as an adaptation, and remake, of the Winston Graham's books. The male lead Aiden Turner is a heartthrob of the day and Canadian and US, as well as GB women have to be held back by security.

Chrys has a wilder alternative to the 'P' beaches named on these beautiful bays. Suggesting that if one can walk comfortably then travel a little further along as if towards Pentewan, on the higher coastal road. Take the turn off towards Trenarren on Blackhead (the dividing outcrop between St Austell and Mevagissey Bays) here one can reaches Hallane Mill. By car, one parks for free at the top of the quaint hamlet and walks down, and through to the sea via the mill which is now a revamped holiday cottage. Again, if the sea is in it's actually a tiny beach, but when out, Chrys suggests climbing or swimming to the right and there are soft sand, and generally very private beach areas.

Seals frequent this small harbour more regularly than the other named popular beaches probably as it's quieter without so many humans. If one does have the luxury, and the privilege to share an area with this beautiful wild creature-leave it alone. They may be inquisitive, but it is not useful for them to get used to humans as many fishermen have a dislike of them. Also as dogs are welcome all year round please make sure the canines don't frighten any wild life and of course to repeat.....pick up your own or any other litter you may find!

The Porthpean environs offer a variety of other 'things to do'. These include; a golf course with a welcoming visitors' cafe; a croquet club that has open days to look out for, and a young person's activity centre. There are also children's and adult hospices at Porthpean, so if one is feeling charitable where better to donate?

Dogs are welcome over the winter months at Porthpean but again check the sea is out for enough sand and rock play room for them.

Pentewan. Pentewan comes from the Cornish 'Bentewyn', meaning 'foot of the radiant stream'. Pentewan is also in this Area of Natural Outstanding Beauty.

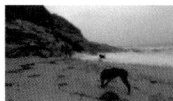

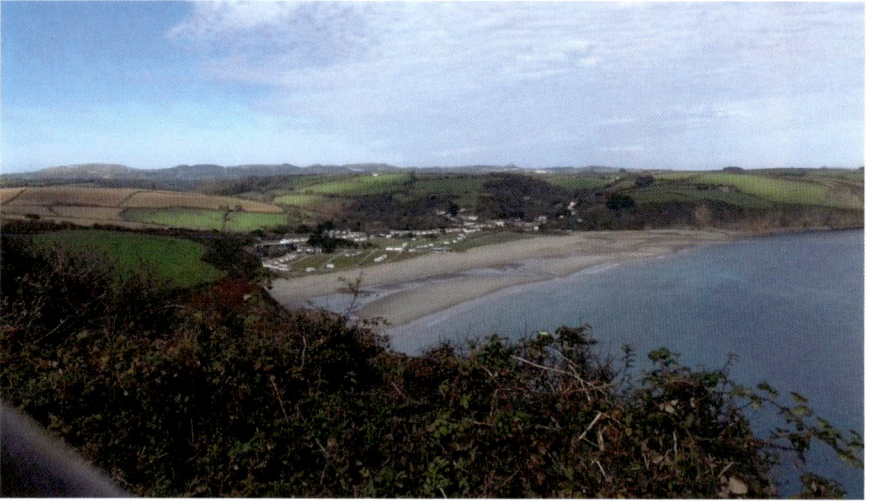

The view from the cliff top path heading towards Mevagissey, looking back towards Pentewan.

Pentewan's exquisite long sandy, east facing beach is split into two; the smaller beach often referred to as the 'Village beach' is separated from the longer beach by a failing and falling old harbour wall. The beaches are additionally divided by the White River that runs from the clay pits near St Austell. Even to this day after a heavy rain, the water runs white with the China Clay silt. Historically, when the industry allowed its waste to run more readily, Pentewan beach was renowned for its' slushy deposits-thankfully now gone.

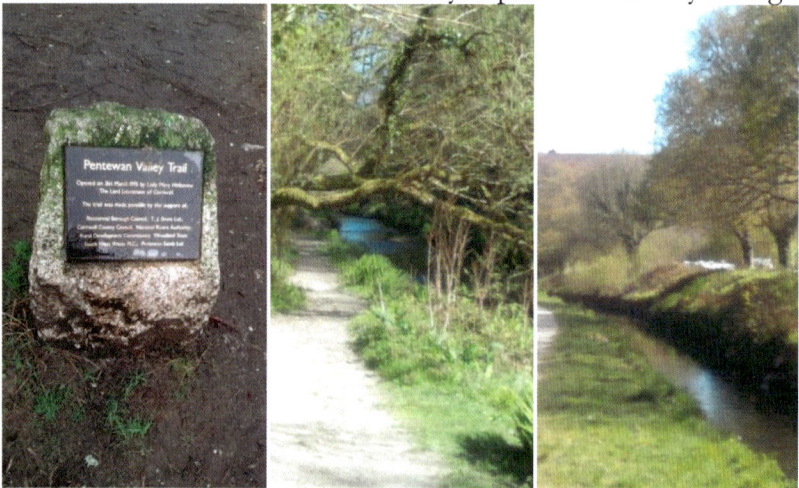

The path following White River joining Pentewan to St Austell now known as the Pentewan Valley Trail; previously the route the railway took.

Both beaches are owned by a local Tremayne family who also own the camping site that lays parallel. that opened its' lawns in 1945. The family has held most of the local land since the Heligan area family led by the Rev. Henry Hawkins Tremayne acquired the land in 1792.One really must find time to peruse the Village information board, it's definitely worth a viewing for historical pictures and interesting information.

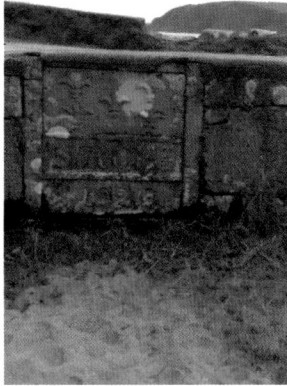

Pentewan Harbour wall, looking south.

The harbour wall was extended to help the pilchard industry and to promote the export of china clay. Tin from the Polgooth mines was also exported, much of which was transported along the Pentewan Valley by a narrow gauge train track that Hawkins also had built and at its peak Pentewan exported a third of the world's china clay! One can see the buckled, rusted remnants of this long gone industrial structureon the outcrop near the start of the Pentewan harbour wall.Ships were unlikely to move empty, as this would waste profits thus Pentewan was also known for importing the much needed coal that was sent in land to be traded. The currently sanded up entrance to the harbour was last used by a cargo ship in 1940.

Chrys moved to this remarkably friendly village, and although she has relocated, still regularly visits Piskey Cove (a favourite). A delight to visit, it offers a wide variety of amazing foods and drinks as well as multiple vegan options they include a shop full of delights and a multitude of ice cream flavours where you can also stay as it's a B&B. Little Bay Café also has many good traditional fayres over looking the harbour and The Ship Inn is a lovely family friendly, St Austell brewery pub offering quiz nights, karaoke, bingo nights and Tim Reynick (for those that know good music) is a Pentewanite, can be seen playing there! The pub also offers a food menu and is (as we write) one of 6 in the finals of a national pub award. This is to say nothing of the village hall film club (fortnightly showings 'out of season' on a Tuesday. Entrance is for a contribution and one can have a hot drink and snack at half time!) The Village hall also hosts the regular meetings of The Old Cornwall Society (OCS), as well as art exhibitions, charity coffee mornings and more. The OCS has given permission for these pictures below as well as the suggestion of two of the local's books on Pentewan; The Past in Pentewan by Robert Evans and Maureen Prettyman. Maureen also wrote Walks in and around Pentewan

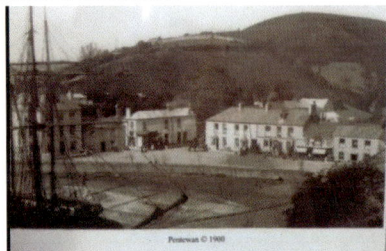

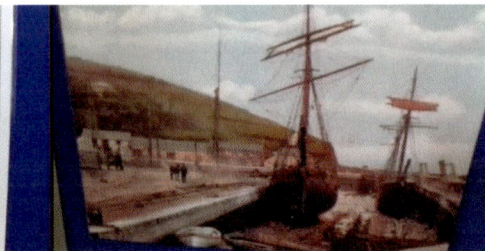

Pentewan was originally occupied in medieval times but built around more extensively when the harbour and the block works were installed, part of which was dramatically unveiled by the sea after a severe storm in early 2018.

During those distant dark aged medieval times; Pentewan was mainly a fishing community-as other coastal villages would have been. It had additional advantages, such as the stone quarry and some tin streaming close by along the river. Of course, the localised agriculture was better than much of Kernow due to the Pentewan valley providing good alluvial soil.

The stream tin mining works and thus industry 'proper' started in 1780. One named, sweetly 'Happy Union' and the other interestingly 'Wheal Virgin'-we cannot imagine those poetic names being applied to industry currently-maybe they should be? Much of the investment was lost due to sea flooding and both were closed by 1874.

Pentewan's quarry produced a superbly attractive and functional building stone named 'elvan', which was volcanically created in the Upper Devonian era. It is therefore a type of igneous called a quartz-porphyry rock, containing large fine grained crystals. This beautifully structured rock adorns many a church entrance including ones in St Austell, Mevagissey and Fowey. Why not see if you can match up and compare rocks you see on the beach and the churches when doing a village visit and a Wild Swim?

Pentewan and Portmelon both have submerged sea forests from when sea levels were far lower than today, though not viewable even at the lowest tides.

Dipping in to the Duchy

Once upon a time this south coast sea was a breeding area for the shallow sea loving grey whale (Eschrichtius robustus); 2 of 7 European fossils were discovered here!! Maybe see if you can find the 3rd fossil when exploring and searching the rock at Pentewan?

The first grey whale to be seen alive by Homo sapiens eyes was in the Atlantic was in 2010. Grey whales tend to be in the Pacific. They are believed to travel through to the Atlantic when the North West Arctic passage opens; so, keep your eyes peeled as this is meant to open more with global warming. There is now (2010s) a marine biological suggestion to re-introduce their breeding to Pentewan. (And, then there really will be no parking spaces in this incredible village!)

It was a 6 meter long Minke whale's horribly decomposing scent that welcomed Chrys and her faithful Lily dog, one cold clear and now rather unfresh morning, when leaving her home on the now fresh water land locked harbour on the 12th January 2015. Minke, the smallest of the whales found in our waters, measuring between 7 and 10 meters when fully grown are not too an unfamiliar Cornish site. For instance a pod of 16 were seen in 2010 in the waters around the Scilly Isles.

So, if one is Wild Swimming here then you may have wonderful company. Chrys once swam within 2 meters of a seal off the Village beach-it came up looked at her with the most beautiful whiskered face and then disappeared. She has also been followed along from Trenarren (as above) to Pentewan by inquisitive seals. (A reminder; to leave them alone; in fact the Marine Strandings Network says if a seal looks at you it is already too disturbed! Please be happy and reminded that 25% of this books profits go to help the MSN)

The beach changes its style, shape and steepness at each tide, and the river meanders across from one end of the longer beach to the Village beach and back-sometimes needing to be humanly re-directed. Be aware of its path, as obviously there will be a drag and possibly invisible undercurrent from its journey through the sea. Easterlies are also a problem here and will create much bigger waves, and possibly a lot of debris in the sea that, may or may not, be visible from above the water level. A good sign that it may not be wise to go in is if one hears the Mevagissey to Fowey (and return) Ferry is not running during the higher season as it usually does. You may like to try this as a super fun ride and note that dolphins are seen on average once per month from aboard!

As hinted at previously this remarkably popular village has the typical emmet (referring to the teeming tourists-meaning 'ants' in Cornish) season difficulty of parking. It is to become a pay and display by Spring 2019. The car parking has two sections but space is really rather limited so again early bird arrival is advisable. Alternatively, one can follow the wonderful Cornish section of the South West Coastal path from surrounding areas, back pack on, and arrive for a swim by foot or choose the cycle path, along the Pentewan Valley. There is of course the option to pay at the campsite which offers limited pay and display car parking. The camp site has a children's play area, an indoor swimming pool, a variety of food outlets, a pub and a shop on site seasonally and provides super Cornish entertainment in its large social area..

Dogs are only made welcome on the beaches at Pentewan between the 1st Sunday in November and the 1st of March each year.

Portmellon-with a brief mentions of Mevaggisey and Gorran Haven.

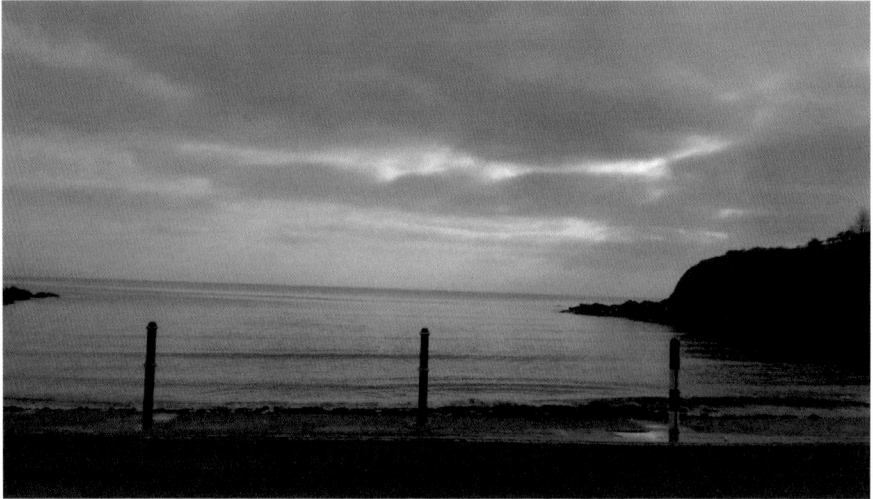

We think that generally when one hears this name one believes it to literally mean melons and per chance imagine a shipwreck releasing yellowy, orange fruit into the local sea: the melons floating, post Wild Water Swim styley in to Portmellon Cove. A little disappointingly to us is that this is not the case; Portmellon's place name means 'cove mill' and was only named this in the 1920s prior to this it was called Portmellin Portmellon is on an area of Devonian rock-remember kellas, and is, as said; part of Cornwall's Area of Natural Outstanding Beauty.

People have though inhabited this area since the 'stone age'; this is not that descriptive as the stone age was an extensive evolutionary phase of human kind stretching back 3.4 million years, but the era was known to end with the advent of metal working. The two defined metal ages; Bronze and Iron started around 8700 and 2000 BCE respectivley (Before the Christian Era) depending on which part of the Earth one was The Metal Ages are deemed to have finished as we came in to the modern era about 600 BCE.

A Bronze Age cemetery was excavated in 1959 which discovered ashes in containers that were 4000 years old. If one follows the Portmellon Valley, you may come across evidence of a Romano/British settlement from the first century AD though evidence for this is undoubtedly hard to find, as is all evidence of Roman occupation west of Exeter.

Portmelon's beautifully amphitheatred, and therefore often very sheltered beach is 150 meters long. It is especially protected and sheltered from the prevailing 'westerlies' (winds) as, again it faces east. The beach is really safe for a great Wild Swim if but only if it's good swimming weather; a potentially necessary repeat of our H&S advice as a human life was lost on the bay only a few years ago. Also, we suggest avoiding sliding down the previous boat launching northerly slope, where the small tributary river runs to the sea; it is barnacled and the climb down a little risky If there's an easterly blowing, the waves crash furiously and violently. In 2018 massive damage was done to the sea fronted houses and the pub during Storm Emma. The clear up took days and the insurance assessors were kept busy for much longer!

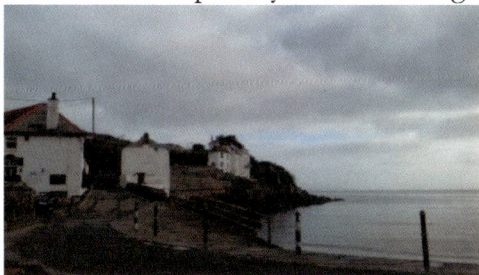

Portmellon looking North towards Mevagissey.

For the more 'risk taking' visitors we recommend waiting for the tide to be fully in, and then, one can jump from the south wall by the pub; The Rising Sun, which boasts locally sourced foods. There used to be a shop run from the pub but this is no longer available.

The aforementioned boat ramp was previously used by the Life boat, stationed here from 1869-1888, before it was moved to Mevagissey. Mevagissey's cholera victims were sent to Portmellon (around 1849) but we haven't found any evidence of the illness re-emerging as the more horror minded, overused imaginations amongst us may fear!

'Meva' as it's colloquially named is over the headland from Portmellon and is a rather picturesque and archetypal Kernow village, adorned with several fantastic watering holes, super shops, great chippies and restaurants.

If exertion is craved, then a swim can be taken further around to the right-facing out to sea, and going along the headland towards Chapel Point. Here one can find tiny, sea accessible only coves to rest and sunbathe in, rocks to climb and dive from and joy, fun, exercise and pleasure to be had.

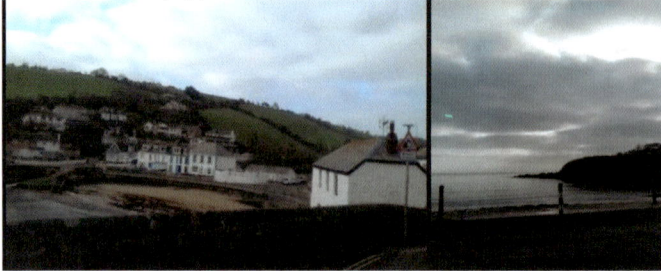

Looking south down in to the village and towards Chapel Point.

As mentioned Portmellon has submerged forest from colder times, when water levels were much lower, when the area now out at sea was fully carpeted with trees. These would have grown during the most recent planetary glacial period that finished roughly 10,000 years; the water was contained in ice sheets elsewhere on the planet. Bog bean and white water lily seeds were also found, suggesting that there was a lake or pool in this area during another geological time though we cannot define this with our research.

Following the coast westward there's another close option for a great swim; it is best reached at low tide and is called Gorran Haven. A jutting rock outcrop delineates where dogs can freely run, off lead all year round to the left away from the harbor area. Gorran Haven is famous for being the first place to catch pilchards (Sardina pilchardus), again using the seining technique; where the fishing net is floated and drops vertically held down by weights. Gorran Haven was, until the eighteenth century anyway, recognized as far more important than the now more active Mevagissey. Both can be reached with delightful coast path promenade, pace or stroll.

Mitchells' boat yard was built in the 1920s to build crafts including Napoleonic warships as well as building 'the Ibis', which was one of the largest ever fishing luggers. The yard is now housing and most boat building has also been transferred to Meva. A lugger is a small sailing boat with sails called lugs, set on two or more masts, an example of which was the 28 ton Windstar that George IV and the young Princess Elizabeth used to travel aboard.

Dogs are welcomed out of season and parking is extremely limited on the surrounding roads. If using the pub and cleaning the beach then it's an option.

6. Trelissick means farm of the leader.

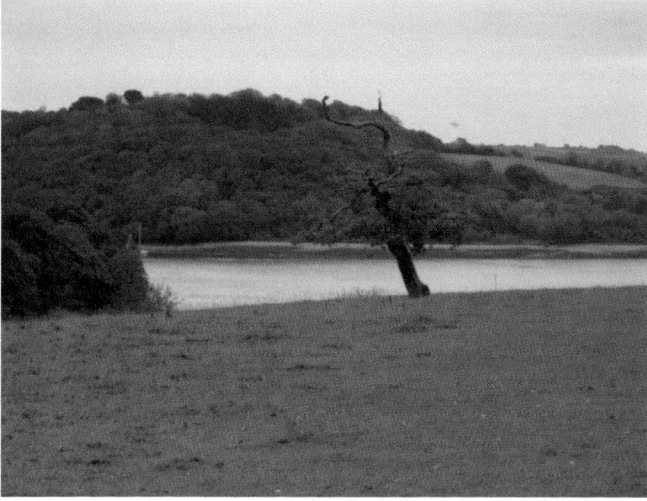

Our final, really rather different, and far further west Wild Swimming venture (for this Book 1, at least) is Trelissick Manor house and gardens near Feock. The area has records of a farm dwelling here since 1275.

The Grade 11 listed building became the property of the national trust in 1955, after having been registered under the Historic Buildings and Ancient Monuments act 1953. It offers free parking for National Trust members-do remember your card which is now scanned (2018).

Trelissick, with its 92 hectares in total provides a real day out for exploring the 10 hectares of gardens and 82 of parklands and woodland; all of which can be used for a warm up or a warm down, before or after your immersion.

One reaches the place we entered the waters (please see pictures) by walking the gentle slopes of a meadow.

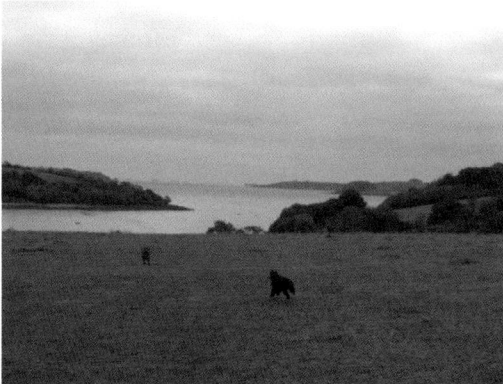

This swim is on the Fal river estuary and is rather different, to our Lostwithiel,

River Fowey swim. The section where we swam is named Carrick Roads; the waters are wide and full. The Fal is a much larger river than the Fowey; from this particular bank one looks out to sea. The Fal is 29km in length and the basin or catchment area covering 223 kilometres.

The river Fal rises on the Goss Moor near to our local town of St Austell and to our aforementioned sea swims, so again literary and alluvial literal connections! As said, this is in the China Clay area, and the first tributaries accumulate near to the village of St Dennis. The Fal continuing its seaward travels running via Grampound, meandering for another 18 km before arriving to sea between Pendennis Point and St Anthony's Head on the English channel. St Dennis is now renowned for being where the 'Cornwall Energy Recovery Centre' is situated; book ahead and you can visit this innovative waste management site (ATL). Six other main tributaries empty into the sea around here, including the Truro River and the entire area is a Nature Reserve of 'international importance'.

The neighbouring harbour of Falmouth is the 3rd largest natural port in the world and has sections with deep water channels. There is frequent controversy between the larger tourist cruise boats who wish to dredge the channels to allow bigger ships in and the conservationists who obviously wish to preserve the natural and rare habitats of many species.

The estuary was formed when the glaciers from the most recent ice age melted away roughly 10,000 years ago; to create a river valley that at some points has a natural depth of 34 meters.

The area was used by the native Celtic peoples of the south west of England for oyster fishing until the Romans came, in fact, most of the Cornish coast has oyster catcheries. Dredging has affected the oyster stocks; oysters take 5 years to grow to maturity and any disturbance takes an awfully long time to heal and mend.

Nowadays giant Russian seafood ships are often blamed, along with the waste from the cargo and tourist ships for the damage being done.

Sail makers and marine engineering industries dotted the shore lines, as well as one might expect the mail boats to-ing and fro-ing from the harbour.

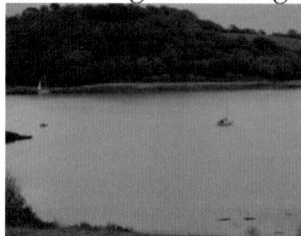

Luxury yachts join the beautiful ocean going liners in these waters, be especially careful of mooring ropes whilst Wild Swimming amongst them.

German 'emmets' are seasonally in abundance. They arrive on vessels coming in to Falmouth harbour, often taking coach tours from here to the familiar and popular Kernow sites. That include, nowadays, where the aforementioned Poldark was filmed, as well as to see where the Rosamund Pilcher series was filmed as this created in the German language.

After World War Two the area was used for vessel scrapping; it's remarkable how adaptable the Fal estuary is. It moves with the times and the needs of the culture it is thrown into. Now that Wild Water Swimming is growing culturally it is, again expanding its uses, one can though imagine that many a Celt or Roman has swum these idyllic waters.

So back to ours, and your adventure at Trelissick: When one arrives at the small beach at the bottom of the garden slope and through the gate, if the sea is in, the temptation is to go in there and then. The trouble is that this section is mud filled shallow area and one may get literally bogged down. We, therefore suggest following in our footsteps and heading along the bank to the left, when facing the sea. There's a path that rises gently, after roughly 50m one finds a slope down to the water that has a super rocky base to launch oneself from. This spot is as a great place to get changed on secure footing without sand getting caught; unexpectedly in any nether regions when disrobing.

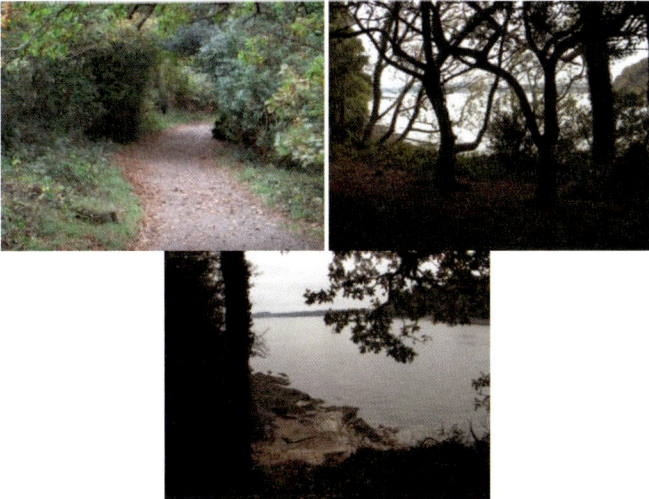

There are boats moored along this area so we suggest not venturing out too far, and definitely being aware of their potential movement as well as of course, and to repeat; looking out for mooring ropes. We delighted in the views and as such an alternative swim, the water is slightly murkier than the sea swims we recommend and much murkier than the Fowey River. Another repetition-in case we haven't rubbed it in enough-please clear up and tidy any non-natural debris you may come across.

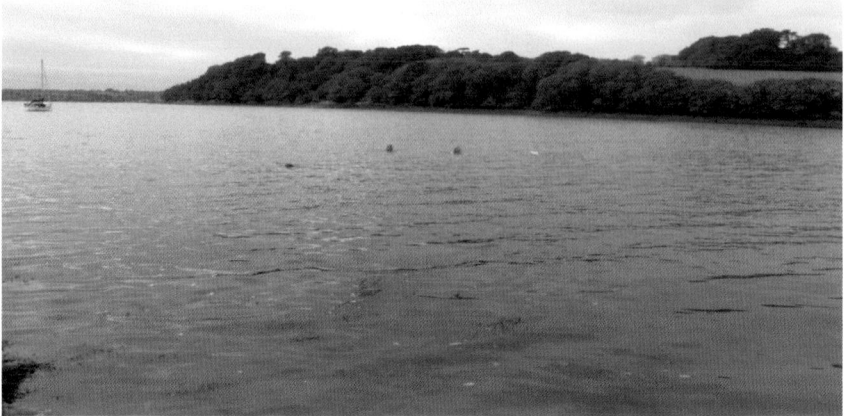

We did not eat at the wonderful café but ate our picnic on the under tree benches provided which was lovely and sociable; not only are the Kernow folk chatty and friendly but holidayers tend to have better moods and even grumpy townies appear to let down their guards!

The café/restaurant does provide a great variety of food and drinks. The second hand book shop, in the courtyard, is a delight and contains books of all types/genres/subjects both factual and fictional. Trelissick House and Gardens additionally offers the delights of an art gallery and sells plants! So we suggest taking your cash.

Here goes as a quick overview; in the 18th century Trelissick was used as a park, in the 19th century when the grounds were planted, followed with the woodland garden. Then, as now, the local wildlife is abundant and exquisite; fallow deer range under skies oft filled with the haunting cries of peregrine falcons and buzzards.

The house was first occupied in 1705 by the Lawrence family. John Lawrence built the current house and laid out the gardens in 1755, with elements of the previous house incorporated. The estate was divided upon his death. The family then entered financial difficulties; it was sold in 1805 to the T.Daniell. He was the son of a tin and copper mine owner as one would perhaps expect for such excessive Cornish wealth. Daniell re-modeled the house in 1825. His fortune also depleted and he was finally declared bankrupt in 1835. Between 1832 and 1844 the property was unoccupied although during this time

Viscount Falmouth of Tregothnan was holding the mortgage.

A man named John Gilbert Davies had inherited the manor of Eastbourne in Sussex, since Cornwall had become a fashionable resort, he bought Trelissick. Gilbert's son, Carew Gilbert Davies then inherited it and extended the buildings after being inspired by much foreign travel.

They owned the house and lands from 1899 until 1927, renting it from 1913 fortunes had again turned and the estate had to be divided in 1927. In 1928 Leonard Daneham Cunliffe, a former governor of the Bank of England, bought the freehold, his stepdaughter later inheriting Trelissick from him in 1937.

The Copelands were the last family to own Trelissick, further developing the gardens even though they were living in Sheffield. The Copeland family moved from the main areas of Trelissick House, and as said many rooms were opened to the public by the National Trust. So you may want to swim, change and, then wander and review the beauty of where you have just swum from the houses' large windows offer the most amazing views.

Protective clothing may need seeking with the aforementioned weather changes in Kernow when venturing on any of the recommended swims but as one is at quite a distance from vehicle access at Trelissick we suggest filling the backpack with weather options!

Enjoy.

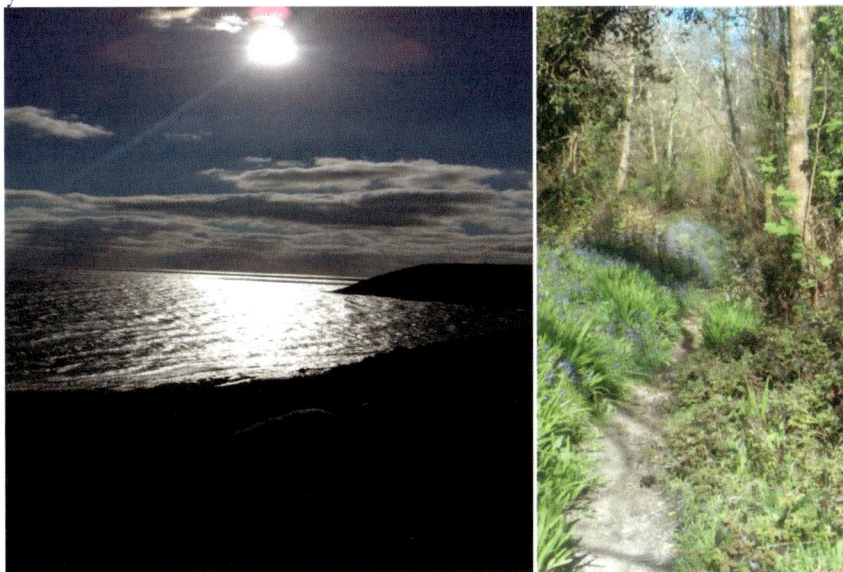

7.Cornish place names;including expressions and pronunciations .

As an introduction to this, out of the way, far end of the land, territory we have a brief guide to Cornish place names and their meanings; translations from Celtic Cornish to English.We also include some commonly heard sayings that you may wish to incorporate into your own dialect; best practiced at the same time as the Kernow accent.

The back pages can be used for you to add any words or expressions you may discover and wish to note. The author would appreciate any additional 'treasures' for future editions☺

Onwards then, linguists……………………………………………………….

You may notice many 'Pols' along your travels this translate as pool.

Equally 'Pen(s)' which can be read as head, end or top.

'Port' or 'Porth' can be read as cove, harbour, or maybe obviously port.

'Bos' is a dwelling.

'Boy' is a friendly and casual term for males and not deemed as condescending as some men may take it 'up country'!

'Carn' a rock pile.

'Car' was once was a fort.

'Chy' becomes 'house' in English.

'Dearovim' or 'Dearover'; These mean "dear of him" and "dear of her", all slurred and blurred into one. It can be said in relation to someone who is sad or struggling or alternatively about a child doing something sweet, as well as a reaction to a shocking story. In other words the meaning is quite variable.

'Dreckly' refers to a rather unspecified time in the future. The Cornish are renowned for being laid back with much of their behaviour and so 'Dreckly' could mean tomorrow, or more likely next week or even next year. Seemingly reflecting the slower pace of life in Kernow.

'Ere' is used to start a gossipy conversation.

'Emmet' as said in the books main text means tourist from the

Cornish word; ant. Basically any foreigner-from across the Tamar that comes and swarms filling the Kernow lanes and waterways!

'Glancing' is being very untidy.

'Goons' are downs.

'Kels' are groves.

'Lan' is a settlement.

'Lowarth' is a garden.

'Lys' a court.

'Maid' refers to women and is a form of endearment not. seen as patronizing!

'Maraz' a market.

'Mel' a mill.

'Men' translates as stone.

Mizzle is a mixture of mist and drizzle.

'Nan' is a valley.

'Park' a field.

'Res' another word for fort.

'Rich' refers to a person's attractiveness; it does not apply to money in this case nor in fact to the flavor of food! Seen as a compliment.

'Rose' a heath.

'Stagged' is when one is overly busy.

'Teasy' is abbreviated from the Kernow speech: "teasy as'n adder" thus implying stroppiness and bad mood.

'Tre' was or is a farm, and

'Wheal' a work or a mine

Fowey is pronounced Foy, Caerhays said Craze and Truro said Trura. We especially like St Austell neing called colloquially Snozzle. There are many more to get your mouth and ear around, most Cornish understand English so, you should be fine☺

8.References, Citations and additional sources of information; Apologies, Thank yous, and contact details for feedback; positive or constructively negative ☺

Special thanks to all the on line sources, TV and Radio programmes, personal conversations and useful societies for providing interesting information and knowledge to us and now you readers.

There are no direct quotes. Maps, graphs and tables were adjusted and renamed but mostly came from Wikipedia-we are aware that this is an open platform and thus, having tried to ask about copyright, have not found any 'right of use' statements.

We refer you to other sources; (excuse the listyness of this); Cornwall in Focus, Cornwall Guide, Beaches in Cornwall, Visit Cornwall, Country Digest, Accessible Countryside for Everyone, Cornwall rivers Project, Mebyon Kernow, Cornwall Council's Website, The National Trust, Royal National Lifeboat Institute, Historic England,www.cornwallcalling.co.uk, The Royal Cornwall Museum, BBC Radio Cornwall, Pirate FM, Heart (Cornwall), St Austell Radio, Yellow Publications who also publish walking and cycling maps, BBC Spotlight, The Guardian, The Daily Mail, The Express, thebeachguide.co.uk Outdoor Swimmer Magazine, Surfers Against Sewage, Outdoor Swimming Society, 3 Bays WildLife Group, Cornwall Ecology and the Cornwall Wildlife Trust.Please remember that 25% of profits from this book goes to their department named The Marine Strandings Network.

You may wish to explore the Wild Swimming subject further via www.wildswimming.co.uk or by searching for the Devon and Cornwall Wild Swimmers.

We apologize in advance if we have provided incorrect information and will be happy to change anything that we agree in future editions.

We also apologize if there is an aspect of Kernow that you may have wished included and we have perchance foolishly left out-again please do contact us and we will see if the book can manage another edit!

Thank you to the environment with all its flora, fauna, geology and varieties of water for the lessons it has taught us, the Kernow people and the way of life for permitting the luxury of becoming authoresses and to all that have helped along the way in any small, medium or large way!

All feedback, ideas, appreciations, constructive criticisms please forward to; czam2003@yahoo.co.uk

If you would be interested Chryseis has a website (currently rather unfinished) promoting her 'therapy' style which can be found at; chryseis.org.uk

If you would like your comment to perhaps be included in later publications or as part of any future publications please do say that with your correspondence.

Again thank you for your time in hopefully adding some width and depth to your appreciation of our wonderful county.

9. Add to list (ATL), and/or sketches and notes.

Dipping in to the Duchy

Dipping in to the Duchy

Dipping in to the Duchy

Dipping in to the Duchy

Dipping in to the Duchy

Dipping in to the Duchy

THE END.

Printed in Great Britain
by Amazon